THE HOME SECURITY SYSTEM AND THE LIPID NEIGHBORHOOD

THE REMIXED 2ND EDITION FOR THE CLINICIAN AND ANYONE ON A MISSION FOR MORE LIPID TUITION

JOSH WAGEMAN
PHD, DPT, MPAS, CLS, CSCS

ISBN: 979-8-9921692-2-5 (paperback)
ISBN: 979-8-9921692-3-2 (ebook)

Interior formatting by *Hannah Linder Designs*

For Mia

Part of me hopes you derive your own creative inspiration from this book someday...but a much bigger part of me just wants you to know that your Dad loves you more than anything.

DISCLAIMER

It's the remixed 2nd edition for the eager clinician
On a demolition mission against systemic attrition
But if you're not a physician and you love erudition
And you're wishin' to bring to realistic fruition
An ammunition acquisition of scientific cognition
A coalition of sedition against the current condition
Then release your inhibition and read this composition!

Oh yeah, and now for the underwhelming, but critical statement from a legality standpoint in a dull, non-hip-hop format:

The opinions expressed in this book are my own and do not represent the dissemination of medical advice. The views expressed herein are not intended to displace or undermine the recommendations of your physician or licensed healthcare professional. This book is intended for enjoyment, edification, and educational purposes only. My opinions do not represent the opinions or strategies of any past or current employer. Also, no artificial intelligence was used to create the manuscript of this book. AI can do many things, but I know it cannot tell the story that you're about to read.

If you enjoyed Peter Attia's *Outlive*, there's something in this book for you.

If you were fascinated by Huxley's *Brave New World*, there's something in this book for you.

If you've been on the verge of bladder incontinence while watching comedian Nate Bargatze, there's something in this book for you.

If you've identified with the plight of King Solomon in *Ecclesiastes*, there's something in this book for you.

If you took Anatomy and Physiology in school and expressed even a modicum of interest in the workings of the human machine, there's something in this book for you.

If you believe that laughter is still oftentimes the best medicine, there's something in this book for you.

And if the first edition of *The Home Security System and the Lipid Neighborhood* left you wanting even more, you might as well start reading!

We're all building castles in the sand.

Some of these castles are barely distinguishable from amorphous dollops of windswept sediment. Some of these castles are utterly sophomoric carbon copies of other beachgoers' prior endeavors. But upon closer inspection, each one of these castles is uniquely crafted and offers some intricate insights into the life of the sculptor.

The Home Security System and the Lipid Neighborhood is my sandcastle. Some might consider it an oasis at the intersection of physiology and literary hedonism. Others might view it as a banal rest stop on the way to more stimulating vacation destinations. But I hope you stop by to appreciate the efforts that have gone into this castle's architecture. I'll even pay for your ticket to join me on the beach if you're particularly picky, prickly, parsimonious, or perhaps all of the above.

And I hope that my sandcastle inspires you to create your own masterpiece. And I hope that my sandcastle is appreciated by at least a few of the passersby. But I know that in the blink of an eye, my sandcastle could be swallowed up by the tide, never to be remembered, vanishing as if it had never existed.

And ultimately, as you build your own sandcastle, I pray that you appreciate the temporal nature of your own life project. Because although your sandcastle will be swept away, your spirit will live on. And your ticket beyond this transient terrestrial sphere has already been purchased by the One who provided your building materials and who gifted you with the capacity to construct.

I hope you join me on that celestial shore one day. I can't buy your ticket...but hopefully I can introduce you to the One who already did.

CONTENTS

PART IV

THE DEEP END OF THE COMMUNITY POOL

THE PRE-GAME SHOW

Uncle Rex was truly a larger-than-life figure. Possessing a disarmingly dazzling smile, twinkling blue eyes, and a booming laugh that echoed throughout the room after one of his self-deprecating jokes, he instantly became the favorite uncle for the entire cluster of impish Wageman cousins. He also had disproportionately short arms for his 6’4” frame, which naturally led to the nickname “T-Rex,” and he embraced this moniker with unquestioned aplomb. Those short arms and admitted gym addiction allowed him to become a local legend on the bench press, and he appeared to be the picture of health. His doctor agreed, stating that his “10-year risk calculator for heart disease barely even registered” and that even though his “bad cholesterol” was moderately elevated, his “good cholesterol” and his “ratio” were completely reassuring. But underneath those chiseled pecs was a coronary tree chock-full of plaque, and our beloved Rex had a near-fatal myocardial infarction at the age of Victimized by a combination of genetics, a complete aversion to cardiovascular exercise, and ignorantly negligent medical advice on the part of his physician, his quality of life was virtu- ally extinct despite surviving the event. And from then on, I dedicated myself to helping others avoid this tragic fate.

Actually, that's really not how it happened, although it would be pretty funny to have an Uncle Rex with short arms (minus the premature coronary disease). I'm an only child, and I have zero uncles on my paternal side of the family. However, terms like "good and bad cholesterol" are erroneous and misleading, 10-year-risk calculators are essentially garbage, and lipid "ratios" generally are superfluous, misinterpreted, and lead to a false sense of security. So at least that was true.

I wish I had an inspiring and humanitarian reason for becoming a Lipid Specialist, but the real story is far less interesting than the fabricated vignette. About 6 years ago, I had a patient cancel her appointment on a cold January day, and whenever I have extra time I generally read various journal articles and scientific literature, which is an obvious red flag for being an incorrigible nerd. So being what I thought was a Biochemistry aficionado, I saw an article with an obnoxiously condescending title...something like "Basics of Lipids and Lipoproteins." I can wax eloquent on glycolytic intermediates all day long, I'm pretty robust on my pentose phosphate pathway, and I almost bought a motorcycle so I could name it Krebs, so I thought to myself, "Lipids...this should be pretty easy." And then I barely understood ANY of what was supposedly a rudimentary review of cholesterol homeostasis. And it annoyed me. And so I decided to embark on a quest to understand everything there is to know about cholesterol, lipids, lipoproteins and the role they play in atherosclerotic cardiovascular disease (ASCVD).

When I was at Yale, one of my classmates asked our program director how we should study for our exams. And he deadpanned, "Just know everything." Nervous chuckles rippled throughout the cohort, and one of the bolder students asked him again. And he said, "No, I'm serious," and walked out. I think most of the class either experienced their first seizure, stroke, or some combination of various cerebral ischemic events that day, but I reflected on his tongue-in-cheek advice. And I liked it...challenge accepted! Because in the quest to "know everything" which will obviously result in inevitable failure, you'll learn a lot. And hopefully on that journey, you'll be able to help some people along the way with the knowledge you've accrued.

My first doctorate was in Physical Therapy, and PT is an awesome profession (I also have a PhD focused on lipid disturbances in Alzheimer's Disease). And although "movement is medicine" and "motion is lotion" and "avoiding inertia sure won't hurt ya" or whatever catch phrase you want to use to make the point that being sedentary is lame, I sort of got bored with orthopedics. The function of the latissimus dorsi hasn't changed since Adam, and it's not like anyone is identifying previously undiscovered musculotendinous units that we all somehow missed for the past few thousand years. But with lipids, I learn new things EVERY DAY, and I consider it a privilege to continually explore the amazing complexities of the human machine.

God gave us bodies to move and minds to think. If you stop moving, you get old. And if you stop thinking, you fall prey to the oft-erroneous sensationalism and GroupThink that pervades merely "trusting consensus." It's hard to know what to believe in the world of cholesterol and lipids, and this book is designed to help you find the proverbial signal amidst all the noise. But not only do I desire to share my realm of expertise with you, I want to share my life with you in a way that resonates more than an impersonal textbook (although I do love textbooks). Because when God gives a gift, he wraps it in a person, and I genuinely care about helping you, whoever you are, NOT have heart attacks, strokes, and dementia. I lack the divine authority to add years to your life, but I believe that I can hopefully help you add "life to your years." Welcome to the Home Security System and the Lipid Neighborhood...it's going to be fun!

INTRODUCING THE HOME SECURITY SYSTEM AND THE LIPID NEIGHBORHOOD

"If you can talk with crowds and keep your virtue
Or walk with kings-nor lose the common touch;
If neither foes nor loving friends can hurt you;
If all men count with you, but none too much;
If you can fill the unforgiving minute
With sixty seconds' worth of distance run-
Yours is the Earth and everything that's in it,
And-which is more-you'll be a Man, my son!"
-Rudyard Kipling, "If"

There are so many things I love about Kipling's majestic poem, but I've always been struck by the concept of "walking with kings but not losing the common touch." Lipids can be incredibly esoteric, and although I am continually fascinated by the intricacy and elegance of biochemical signaling pathways, I also deeply value human interaction. And I REALLY need friends, because as my wife can attest, I'm basically good at about 3 things and am an abject disaster at pretty much everything else. I didn't even own a bed until we got married, instead preferring to crash on various beanbag chairs and couches as I nomadically and somewhat aimlessly navigated various strata of academia. I strive to have a truly regal understanding of human physiology, but if I can't communicate these concepts in a relatable manner, then I've lost that all-important common touch that could otherwise leave an indelibly positive imprint on someone's life. And so as I have invested myself in the study of cholesterol homeostasis, this mantra has served as a valuable compass to help me from teetering over the precipice of unintelligible erudition.

So, for everyone who **DOESN'T** want to have heart attacks, strokes, and dementia, I want you to have a **GREAT HOME SECURITY SYSTEM** and **LIVE IN A SAFE LIPID NEIGHBORHOOD**. Your Home Security System has 4 basic pillars:

1. **Normalize blood sugar (parameters of glucose metabolism).**
   a. No one ever said, "Boy I wish I was more insulin resistant!"
2. **Keep blood pressure normal**
   a. Despite what my patients would tell me, 220/120 is not "normal for you" unless normal is having strokes every other week.
3. **Keep inflammation low**
   a. Life is not better inflamed than non-inflamed.
4. **Don't smoke (or other drugs...drugs are bad).**
   a. I think they still teach the kids that...maybe.

Phrased another way, the 4 essential pillars of the Home Security System basically represent your **ENDOTHELIAL FUNCTION**. The endothelium is a layer of cells that lines your blood vessels and adapts to various environmental stimuli, maintaining an optimal physiologic milieu so you can feel protected against any metabolic miscreants.

But then your **NEIGHBORHOOD is your LIPID PANEL**, because every **<u>LDL PARTICLE</u>** (it really isn't the mass of LDL cholesterol) is **a <u>POTENTIAL CRIMINAL</u> that can BREAK IN to your PHYSIOLOGIC HOUSE**. As you will learn later, these particles are mailmen, but these mailmen can sometimes run their trucks into your arterial wall. And the **Lp(a) (pronounced el-pee-little-ay) particles,** if you picked the wrong parents with that genetically determined lipoprotein, are the **POTENTIAL FELONS** (since, per particle, they are~6.5x as likely to cause vascular disease than your run-of-the-mill LDL particle).

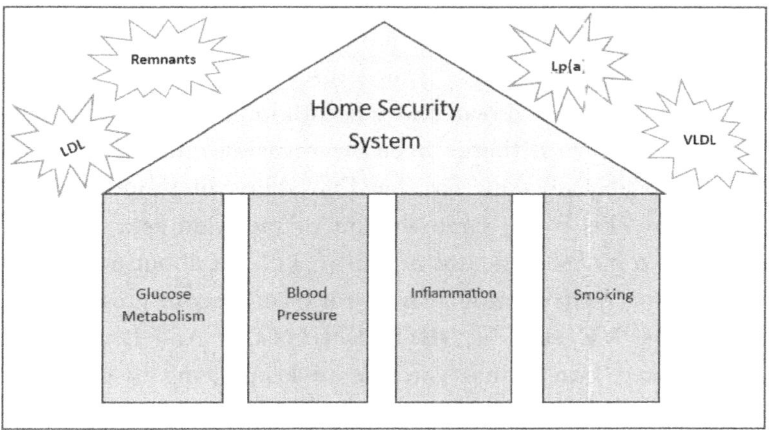

Figure 1: The Home Security System and Lipid Neighborhood. The 4 pillars of the Home Security System representative of endothelial integrity are optimization of glucose metabolism, normalizing blood pressure, keeping inflammation low, and not smoking. Every ApoB-containing lipoprotein is potentially a "criminal" that could infiltrate the neighborhood. Instead of "delivering the mail" of triglycerides to muscle and fat cells, the mailman "runs his truck into the artery wall," which is the initiating event in atherosclerosis. The vast majority of these particles under normal conditions are LDL particles, although remnants and Lp(a) particles can be particularly atherogenic.

So, how's your Home Security System? How's the Neighborhood you're living in? Pretty much any health care professional will test for the aforementioned biomarkers (aside from maybe Lp(a) until they meet me and we talk about it). But people don't live on paper....so how can we determine if you have been "broken into?" It may appear as if you're living in a rough inner-city neighborhood based on your bloodwork, but do we have any diagnostic imaging tests that can better inform us? We do!

The catchphrase I use to address this topic is **"Got plaque? Get a CAC!"** CAC stands for CORONARY ARTERY CALCIUM SCAN. It's the **"colonoscopy of the heart without the nasty pregame show."** (If you've had a colonoscopy and done the bowel prep, you understand how that process temporarily ruins your social life and potentially destroys your bathroom). But basically it tells you if you've been broken into or not, since calcified plaque in your coronary arteries is a late finding in the process of atherosclerosis development. All you have to do is lay down, take a breath in, and then a low-dose CT scan tells you if there's been an intrusion into your arterial abode. (To allay any concerns that I'm asking you to move to the Chernobyl, this is the same amount of radiation as a mammogram at 0.6 milliseverts...for reference, you get about 6 milliseverts per year just existing). So if you have a score greater than zero, **YOU'VE BEEN BROKEN INTO.** And if you have been broken into, would you like to keep living in the same neighborhood in which you've been the victim of a crime, or would you prefer to move to a nice, safe gated community with fewer criminals? This is where various lipid-lowering medications come into play. Put another way, if you have ANY plaque in your coronaries, would you prefer that plaque stable or unstable? And would you like to potentially further stabilize that plaque AND potentially reduce the volume of plaque in your arteries? Is that even possible? It actually is, and we have tools in our therapeutic toolbox to accomplish just that!

If you stop reading here, you'll at least have received more education regarding cardiovascular disease prevention than most medical programs offer. But stick with me, and we will continue to add color to this foundational metaphor as we further explore the elements of the Home Security System and the Lipid Neighborhood.

THE COMMUNITY POOL OF THE LIPID NEIGHBORHOOD

In renovating the Lipid Neighborhood, I have added a Community Pool designed for Deep Dives of Physiology. And maybe you aren't currently confident in your ability to swim; that's totally fine, and the rest of the book will equip you with the foundational skills to navigate the Deep End when you're ready. And maybe you just want to dip your toe in the waters of complex biochemistry...that's ok, too. And maybe the last time you attempted a deep dive you belly flopped into a morass of intolerably convoluted scientific jargon and are still sore...there are plenty of other activities in the Lipid Neighborhood that will help you move on from those past traumas. And maybe you're not a "water person" because of an emergency Code Brown evacuation of your kiddie pool when you were a child...or maybe you were the cause of the Code Brown evacuation (this is a safe space, you can admit it). Regardless, you don't HAVE to take the plunge into the wonderful depths of knowledge that the Community Pool possesses...but when you do muster up the courage, I doubt you'll regret it!

Rules of the Pool

There is no lifeguard on duty at the Community Pool, but I want to ensure the safety of all the participants, so I have eliminated two potential hazards from the resort. There will be no ducks. And there will be no Essential Oils. Let me explain.

Although baby ducks are inarguably cute (and I've heard their cuteness has even been proposed as a remedy for most etiologies of existential angst), I have a personal distrust of pool-dwelling mallards. When I was playing college baseball, our team was playing a series down in California. For some reason, I decided to swim in the hotel pool prior to our game, which was unusual for several reasons. One, I'm a terrible swimmer (I entered a triathlon once and after the swim portion I was in 185th place out of 200 people...the people beating me were much closer to Michael Moore in physique than Michael Phelps). And number two, I don't even like swimming...but there I was, splashing around like a Magikarp in a Southern California pool (for those who don't know, Magikarp is the most useless Pokemon in existence...my daughter is currently obsessed with Pokemon). And immediately after I exited the pool, a flock of ducks descended into the water. Perplexed and concerned, I asked the hotel manager if this was a normal occurrence, and he (not so) reassuringly replied, "Oh yeah, those ducks just live in the pool." I then asked about chlorination, but he didn't seem familiar with that word.

So the next day on the long bus ride home, I ended up needing my own personal emesis bag and multiple stops at gas stations were made on my behalf...and those pit stops were not merely to get some snacks. I'm pretty sure I played a prominent role in initiating the policy of placing "Restrooms for Customers Only" signs on these establishments. Things continued to get worse, and I singlehandedly put a premature ending to our locker room team meeting with the sheer volume of my exploits as I lived the "Laxative Retribution" scene from Dumb and Dumber. I eventually got a ride to the emergency room and it turns out that I had acquired amoebic dysentery from those ducks. Those birds may give you a warm fuzzy feeling when you look at them, but you just can't trust them...that warm, fuzzy feeling might actually be the start of a protozoal infection.

And there will be no Essential Oils. One time after a perfect storm of a 95-degree day, a Spartan Race at altitude, and ill-advised tinkering with my thyroid dosing regimen resulted in an episode of rhabdomyolysis, my wife decided to draw up a warm Epson salt bath. This seemed like a sweet idea, since I couldn't really walk and my leg muscles were spasming with such amplitude that our dog had refused to sit on my lap.

Unbeknownst to me, a friend had given my wife some Essential Oils and one of those diffuser gadgets that propagates the aroma throughout the house. And my wife thought it would be a perfect opportunity to employ the lemony fragrance of the Essential Oils; this would be an ideal complement to the soothing Epson salt bath for her crippled husband. But instead of using the diffuser, she simply dumped the ENTIRE BOTTLE into the bathtub. Path of least resistance, baby...that's the Wageman Way!

Unfortunately, she completely ignored the "WARNING: Not for Topical Use" label on the bottle. So after dragging my debilitated body like a three-legged grasshopper to the bathtub and plopping myself in, I noticed an unusual tingling sensation after about 45 seconds. And that tingling soon metamorphosed into the full-fledged perception that MY SKIN WAS BEING SCALDED. Resembling the love child of an amateurishly-peeled orange and a lobster, I forgot about my previously incapacitated legs and hobbled to the shower to douse my second-degree burns in deliciously cold water. She felt bad, and we laughed about it later as she helped debride my blistered integument. Maybe topical use of Lemony Zest Essential Oils is the real cure for statin-associated myalgias...it'll burn you so severely that you'll forget about everything else.

So no ducks. And no Essential Oils. I want your experience at the Community Pool to be free of gastrointestinal explosions and dermatological trauma.

PART I

THE HOME SECURITY SYSTEM

PILLAR 1: NORMALIZE BLOOD SUGAR

"Control your insulin, control your life."
-Josh Wageman

When I was in high school, I was writing a critical analysis of Dickens' *A Tale of Two Cities*. It was, in some ways, the best of essays, but also the worst of essays (see what I did there?), but as I was weaving my linguistic tapestries, I fashioned a particularly rich sentence practically pregnant with pathos. So I referenced myself after the quote; I wanted to make sure that credit was properly ascribed, and upon completion of the paper, I turned it in. A couple of days later, my teacher called me up to her desk and candidly asked me, "Did you just quote yourself here?" and, of course I unabashedly claimed authorship. "You can't do that!" she exclaimed, and I ended up getting a few points deducted from my grade. Apparently that sort of thing is frowned upon, but I think that since I'm now the one writing the book, I can take liberties that never would have been possible in Sophomore Honors English. So yeah, I've been stressing the importance of optimizing insulin for a LONG time.

So what is insulin? Most people are aware that it lowers your blood sugar (glucose), which is true. ("Sugar" and "glucose" will be used interchangeably throughout this chapter). And you may know that it's produced by the beta cells of the pancreas (if you're really savvy you might know the pancreatic alpha cells also produce glucagon, and if you're really wanting that completely pointless gold star you might even mention delta cells and somatostatin). But insulin is really a storage hormone. When you eat, it goes up, and when you haven't eaten for a while, it should go down. After you eat, you're in storage mode, so insulin rises, and then when you shift to burning mode, insulin should be pretty low. Our bodies are supposed to shift seamlessly from fasted to fed states and then we all live happily ever after.

However, most Americans, particularly those partaking in the Standard American Diet (no coincidence that acronym is SAD), are perpetually in storage mode...even when fasting, insulin levels are CHRONICALLY HIGH. This is a MASSIVE PROBLEM and is often referred to as INSULIN RESISTANCE, which is really an issue with fuel partitioning, or if you want to sound like a scholar, SUBSTRATE UTILIZATION.

Essentially, there are 3 sources of fuel that we can utilize to generate the energy necessary for life. These include FAT, GLUCOSE, and PROTEIN. Although protein is of critical importance for preservation of muscle mass and ketones can also be used as an alternative fuel source, for our current conversation of energy production we will focus on FAT and GLUCOSE. **FAT is basically your body's SAVINGS ACCOUNT**... even those of us who are very lean have a virtually unlimited supply of fatty acids. And really, this is the fuel you ought to be using right now as you're sitting there reading this book, at least below the brain. **GLUCOSE is like DOLLAR BILLS**, and when you need to generate energy quickly, which is dictated by the intensity of your activity, you

> **What about protein?**
>
> Protein is a lot like metal. You can use metal, like pieces of flint, to create a fire, but it's not a great long-term solution. Metal is best used for making tools. In the same way, protein is not a great fuel source for energy production; it's best used for building muscle, an essential tool that keeps your metabolic fire burning brightly. However, paper (glucose) and wood (slow-burning fat) are the primary fuel sources that generate energy (ATP) and keep your fire burning. (Credit to Dr. Andy Galpin, from whom I first heard this excellent metaphor).

use the dollar bills. **HOWEVER, most people are OVERLY RELIANT on the dollar bills and NEVER ACCESS THEIR SAVINGS ACCOUNT**...even when the activity doesn't demand rapid energy production. Instead, they fumble around in their wallet, trying to extract some dollar bills... and then they drop their wallet and don't end up using the dollar bills OR their savings account. That's insulin resistance, which over time leads to impaired glucose levels, then prediabetes, then full-blown Type 2 diabetes. But it's all a continuum, analogous to the absurdity of being "mostly pregnant;" you're either insulin resistant or you're not. It's just a matter of how far along you are.

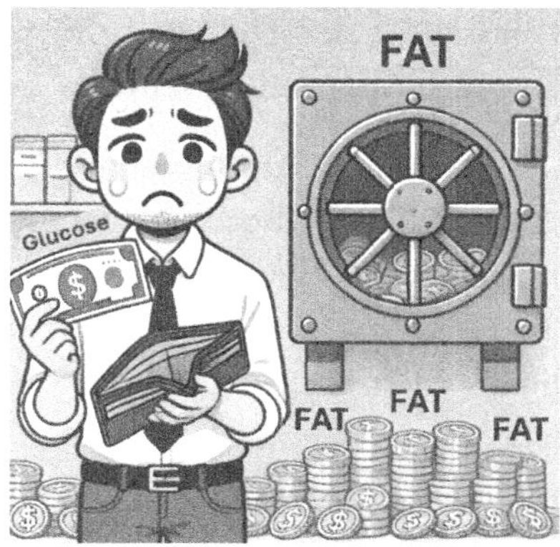

Figure 2: The Bankruptcy of Insulin Resistance. Instead of accessing the virtually unlimited "savings account" of fatty acids, most people are overly reliant on the "glucose dollars," which inevitably results in a failure to pay the energy bill.

Dr. Jason Fung describes insulin resistance rather poignantly and likens the body's fat cells to little suitcases. Insulin comes along and via the action of something called lipoprotein lipase (LPL), shoves the clothes (whatever calories you just ate packaged into triglycerides) into your suitcases. And if insulin needs to specifically put glucose into those suitcases, it must use an "access code" called the GLUT4 transporter to unlock the cellular satchel. But over time, the suitcases start to get full. Your subcutaneous fat increases, and depending on your genetics, you may have more or less room in your subcutaneous fat suitcases...but you keep eating. And insulin levels continue to rise, recruiting more and more insulin friends to try to jam those clothes into your packed suitcases...and then one day you are completely out of room. Moreover, your GLUT4 cellular access code is denied... your suitcases are full AND you're locked out! So insulin drapes the excess caloric clothes around your liver, pancreas, heart, and other organs (fatty liver sounds gross, but fatty heart should strike you as particularly nasty...and fat around your heart is one of the strongest predictors of having a cardiac event). And that's when everything goes completely wrong...you're starving in the midst of plenty, and the risk of dying from pretty much any cause (other than true starvation) essentially goes through the roof.

I'm not kidding...the risk of all-cause mortality is about 50% higher in people who have elevated insulin levels EVEN IF BLOOD SUGARS ARE NORMAL. And then if your blood sugar AND insulin are high, your risk of dying goes up by a mere 232%!

Just in case you're not convinced, I'll briefly give you a few more reasons to prioritize this all-important concept of glucose and insulin optimization.

Blood Pressure

Under normal circumstances, insulin is a VASODILATOR, meaning your blood vessels widen and blood flow is streamlined. This is due, in large part, to insulin's activation of something called endothelial nitric oxide synthase (eNOS). BUT, when someone is insulin resistant, instead of activating eNOS, insulin upregulates a VASOCONSTRICTOR called endothelin-1. And literally the opposite of what is supposed to happen results, contributing to increased risk of hypertension.

Cancer

At least 13 different cancers are directly influenced by diabesity, and this is in large part due to insulin's role as a MITOGEN (think "mitosis" and cell replication) in a cellular pathway called MAPK (couldn't resist). It also activates a "growth signal" called Mechanistic Target of Rapamycin Complex 1 (mTORC1). Basically, insulin drives PROTEIN SYNTHESIS, which is good if you're lifting weights (and bodybuilders will often use exogenous insulin for its anabolic effects when they're trying to get as huge as possible). But if you're not aggressively pulling the exercise lever and you've got a bunch of extra insulin around, insulin often turns on the kind of protein synthesis and growth signals you DON'T want, leading to tumor development...and once that fire has started, excess glucose often further fans the flame.

Obesity and Heart Disease

Insulin also turns on genes associated with something called de novo lipogenesis, which basically just means you create even more fat...just what you need! And since you're not using your savings account, the fat continues to accumulate in and around your organs! And another normal function of insulin is to prevent your fat cells from liberating their stored triglycerides in a process called LIPOLYSIS. But, unable to prevent this, even more fat floods back to the liver, leading to even more fat production in the liver itself and additional packaging of those triglycerides into LIPOPROTEINS (a little foreshadowing for the Lipid Neighborhood discussion that will ensue in the near future). And since there's no available storage space in your suitcases, these cholesterol and triglyceride-laden particles often make their way into your arterial wall, one of the reasons why people with diabetes have a 2 to 4-fold risk of dying from heart disease.

Fatty Liver

As mentioned, a common consequence of insulin resistance has historically been referred to as non-alcoholic fatty liver disease (NAFLD), but has recently come to be known as metabolic-associated steatohepatitis (MASH). I actually like MASH, given that if you're shaped like a potato, your liver is probably swimming in fatty gravy. But while we're on the topic, there is an interesting new medication on the horizon for MASH called pegozafermin, an FGF21 analogue. FGF21, which stands for Fascinating and Greatly beFuddling (actually it's fibroblast growth factor 21) acts via both direct and central mechanisms, increasing fatty acid oxidation in the liver and improving glucose homeostasis. (FGF21 is also known as the "Sweet Tooth Gene" since variants in FGF21 seem to predispose individuals to craving saccharine treats). In early studies pegozafermin seems to be effective at both reducing liver fat and reducing serum triglycerides...stay tuned! But while you're waiting, might as well start becoming less insulin resistant.

Inflammation

Even your macrophages, your body's infection fighters, are supposed to rely on the fatty acid savings account if they're going to effectively do their jobs in neutralizing bacteria and viruses. There are two main types of macrophages: M1 (which are pro-inflammatory and make things worse) and M2 (which are anti-inflammatory and help clean up messes). M1 macrophages predominate in people who are insulin resistant and they rely on SUGAR for fuel, whereas the good anti-inflammatory macrophages are fueled by fat. Interestingly, medications such as GLP-1 receptor agonists like Semaglutide shift your macrophages from M1 to M2, and that's why we see a significant decrease in inflammatory markers like C-reactive protein (hs-CRP) in those clinical trials.

Alzheimer's Disease

Although the brain can utilize alternative fuel sources such as ketones or glucose-derived lactate, its preferred fuel is glucose. This is why if you decided to not eat for the next couple of weeks, your blood sugar would regulate right around 60-70 mg/dL; this is because your liver, via a process called gluconeogenesis, will make its own sugar and it will freely diffuse across the blood brain barrier to supply the brain with precious glucose. Some of the earliest signs in asymptomatic individuals who will later go on to develop Alzheimer's is underutilization of glucose in the brain, and people with pre-existing Alzheimer's show decreased uptake of glucose in the brain as well. Quite predictably, individuals with diabetes have a markedly elevated risk of succumbing to dementia, which you may have heard referred to as Type 3 diabetes.

Kidney Disease, Neuropathy, and Retinopathy

Have you ever wondered why people with diabetes get NEPHROPATHY (kidney disease), NEUROPATHY (can't feel their feet or if they can, it burns) and RETINOPATHY (basically going blind)? Well, these issues, which are referred to as

Insulin in Type 1 Diabetes

In a relatively lean person, the normal pancreas makes between 18 and 40 units per day. However, people with Type 1 diabetes obviously need exogenous insulin to normalize blood sugars and not die. But I've had patients come to me on 100, 200, even 750 units of insulin per day...that's INSANE (and the gal who came to me on 750 units had unfortunately, and not coincidentally, had 4 heart attacks as well). So when too much insulin is employed for those with Type 1, these people end up getting DOUBLE DIABETES, adding profound insulin resistance to their issue of genetic insulin deficiency. And that results in an exponentially increased risk of cardiovascular complications.

MICROVASCULAR COMPLICATIONS, are uniquely due to the toxicity of high blood sugars. A blood sugar of 180 is a poisonous threshold incompatible with normal cellular processes, but our bodies are pretty phenomenal at doing damage control. So in an effort to mitigate the sugar toxicity, your body converts the excess glucose into SORBITOL. But this isn't a very good solution, since sorbitol is really bad news as well! Thankfully, the enzyme sorbitol dehydrogenase, which converts sorbitol to fructose, comes to the rescue, and although excess fructose can be problematic in the long-term, you'll live to fight another day. Crisis temporarily averted! Except in the kidneys, nerves, and eyes...those organs lack sorbitol dehydrogenase, so that sorbitol accumulates and wrecks your ability to see, pee, and fee(l). (That was a stretch). Giving insulin to people with diabetes to better control blood sugars does reduce these microvascular issues...but insulin certainly doesn't help reduce the risk of heart attacks and strokes, which are sort of important events to avoid.

How Can I Check for Insulin Resistance and Assess My Parameters of Glucose Metabolism?

At this point, hopefully we are all intent on NOT being insulin resistant. Some people do have more of a genetic predisposition to insulin resistance, but these susceptibilities can be overcome with early identification and intervention. Anytime we are attempting to measure these parameters of your Home Security System or Lipid Neighborhood, we employ BIOMARKERS, which are often BLOOD-BASED. There are SO MANY blood tests you could get to assess every nook and cranny of your metabolic milieu, and aside from the practicality of cost considerations, you have to ask yourself with ANY biomarker or diagnostic imaging test these critical questions:

1. **Do I understand the results?**
2. **Are the results actionable?**

I would often have patients ask me to run every test under the sun (these were usually the same patients with college-ruled notebooks containing lists of these lab tests along with a duffel bag of all the supplements they were also taking). And since I'm not a jerk, I'd go through all the tests and all the supplements and explain the utility (or not) of each diagnostic test and supplement...this is also why I made about $14 an hour when I was in clinical practice. But anyway, after a thorough analysis and explanation of all the wonderful and often superfluous things, if they still wanted me to run blood tests assessing the hydroxylated derivatives of their adrenocortical steroid hormones, I would do it. And if they wanted to see if somehow their MTHFR genotype had changed, I would run it. And if they wanted to continue taking 3 different forms of CoQ10 dosed at 4-hour intervals, hopefully they were getting one of those liquid ones that actually taste super good.

So in checking for insulin resistance, could you get an oral glucose tolerance test? Sure. Could you wear a continuous glucose monitor? If you have diabetes, you absolutely should. Should you check your 1,5 anhydroglucitol and/or fructosamine? (Yes, those are actual tests that assess short-term glucose levels/variability and I have actually ordered those in a few situations). There are SO MANY OPTIONS out there, but there are several common tests that can actually be quite useful and actionable when assessing your parameters of glucose metabolism. So here they are:

1. **Hemoglobin A1c** (HbA1c)- this represents the average blood glucose for the last 3 months.
2. **Fasting glucose** (which comes as part of a complete metabolic panel, or CMP).
3. **Fasting insulin** (a separate test)
   a. If you are on insulin and have Type 2 diabetes, you can check a c-peptide. Your insulin level will be affected by the exogenous insulin you're taking, but c-peptide is a protein that is only produced at the same time your pancreas makes its own insulin. This is a way to determine if your beta cells are "burnt out" or not. And if not, it means that, with the right combination of

C-peptide: Beyond Identifying Beta Cell Reserve

Savvy clinicians can also utilize c-peptide to assess for hyperinsulinemia. C-peptide can only be produced when the pancreas makes insulin, and both insulin and c-peptide are made in equal amounts. However, insulin has some things to do in the liver (like storing glycogen and putting the brakes on gluconeogenesis), so not all of it makes it into the bloodstream. Conversely, c-peptide is simply released into the blood stream and actually has a little bit longer half-life. So if you're using c-peptide in lieu of fasting insulin, shooting for a goal of <1.3 ng/mL is good as long as blood sugars are concurrently normal.

medication catalysts and lifestyle modification, you can completely get off of your insulin! I had one gentleman who was on 420 units of insulin when he came to me and his HbA1c was still 9.1 (not really doing the job...the threshold for diabetes is 6.5). But his c-peptide was sky-high, and with a little Semaglutide, some specific dietary coaching, and myself and his family cheering him on, he was able to get off ALL HIS INSULIN, drop 70 pounds, and get his HbA1c down to 6.2! But more importantly, he was riding his bike with his wife and able to be a better father, employee, and friend; he got off his insulin and got his life back, which is amazing.

b. More commonly, you'll see a young person with a HbA1c of 4.8, fasting glucose of 80 (totally normal), but a fasting insulin of 30! (For reference, my fasting insulin is generally below 2 and I get flagged as a potential Type 1 diabetic), and that's a common finding in very insulin-sensitive, lean people. But with the combination of fasting insulin and fasting glucose, you can calculate what's called a Homeostatic Model Assessment of Insulin Resistance (HOMA-IR). If you multiply fasting insulin by fasting glucose and divide by 405, you get a value that, if over 2, means you're VERY INSULIN RESISTANT. So in the above example, that patient would be told she's in perfect shape since her glucose is below 100 and her HbA1c is quite low...but her HOMA-IR is 5.9! Definitely need to cut the soda, stop the Doritos, and learn to deadlift, because insulin resistance is just the earliest sign of inevitable progression to impaired fasting glucose, prediabetes, and Type 2 diabetes down the line. But more importantly, it shows that your Home Security System is already significantly compromised.

c. You'll also obtain some additional useful information from that CMP, which includes your various electrolytes, liver function tests (which is a bit of misnomer, but this includes your AST and ALT... many reasons these can be elevated, but very commonly due to fatty liver...which is usually due to INSULIN RESISTANCE), and kidney function measured by estimated glomerular filtration rate (eGFR). And since an eGFR even below 75 (they don't even say you have chronic kidney disease, or CKD, until you're under 60) is associated with croaking off from any cause...and we already know how blood sugar fluctuations can destroy your kidneys...it's pretty important to make sure those kidneys are stayin' in the flow.
    i. Wishing to instill an appreciation for the kidney in my daughter, I bought her a stuffed plush kidney and named it Zac...Zac Nephron...she didn't really get it, but I did earn a courtesy chuckle out of my wife.

The Solution to Insulin Resistance/Prediabetes/Diabetes (or better yet, preventing it all)

So what is the solution? Well, if the caloric clothes are draped around your LIVER and PANCREAS, remove the clothes. Unpack your subcutaneous fat suitcases and make room for your nutritional wardrobe. You retrain your body to use its savings account. You restore insulin sensitivity. Your GLUT4 access code is renewed. And guess what? Even Type 2 diabetes is reversible! If necessary, certain medications like GLP-1 receptor agonists and SGLT2 inhibitors can help catalyze the restoration of insulin sensitivity rather than serving as a band-aid; those classes of medications actually reduce the risk of cardiovascular events in contrast to exogenous insulin. And better yet, if you take a preventive approach to substrate utilization, you can essentially stop worrying about virtually everything that could destroy your physiologic milieu. So how do you do it? Brace yourself...the solution I'm offering may very well elicit skepticism about my multiple advanced degrees.

1. **Get good sleep**
2. **Don't eat crap**
3. **Move**
4. **Keep it up throughout your whole life**

I know, earth-shattering stuff, and I get the sense you'd like me to elaborate. So I will...a little.

1. The quickest way to insulin resistance is sleep deprivation. One of the most fascinating studies I've ever read was one in which they enrolled college kids at the height of their mitochondrial powers, completely devoid of insulin resistance (which was even measured with an oral glucose tolerance test). They forced one group to sleep less than 4 hours a night, and the other group just slept like they normally would. And after JUST 5 DAYS, half of the sleep-deprived group had levels consistent with prediabetes on their repeat oral glucose tolerance test. It takes a long time of blitzing the buffet and being simultaneously sedentary to arrive at the undignified throne of prediabetes/diabetes, but if you don't sleep, you don't even need a week. Crazy.

2. Diet is a profoundly polarizing topic that inevitably winds up provoking a religious tribalism. There are multiple diets that one can employ to achieve metabolic health. And what is "eating crap," you ask? Well, I'll just say that no one looks at a corn dog and thinks to him or herself, "Yes, I'm consciously making a healthy choice

here." If it seems unhealthy, it probably is. And you could get super granular and micromanage your macronutrients. And you could use a Continuous Glucose Monitor (CGM), even if you're not diabetic (this always cracks me up...these individuals come in two basic flavors. They either will use the CGM to make the ground-breaking "discovery" that the Costco muffin they ate spiked their blood sugars...the other camp will ironically stress out so much about minor variations in their blood sugars that they will inadvertently start trending in the wrong glycemic direction). Or you can do this:

a. Prioritize protein
b. Eat real food
c. Avoid processed, refined-carb garbage
    i. And that will probably work.

3. Movement entails a combination of aerobic exercise and resistance training. And without getting into the deep weeds of strength and conditioning, here are a few concepts that can provide you some basic guidance.
    a. When you're doing aerobic exercise, sitting on the recumbent bike watching Netflix probably won't cut it. You should be able to hold a conversation, but whoever is listening to your conversation should be able to tell that you're exerting yourself. And that's a good rule of thumb

If It's Muscle You LACK, You Probably have CAC

In keeping with the axiom, "No one ever said I wish that I was weaker," low muscle mass is independently associated with both presence AND progression of coronary artery calcium (CAC). So if it's MUSCLE YOU LACK, then you PROBABLY HAVE CAC! Better go pick up some heavy things!

for engaging in what you've probably heard referred to as "Mitochondrial Zone 2" aerobic exercise.

i. While we're here, I would be remiss if I didn't briefly discuss the mitochondria. Everyone can smugly identify the mitochondria as the "powerhouse of the cell," and I'm pretty sure this is the only factoid that most people can regurgitate from 7th grade Biology. But really, as long as there's enough oxygen around, any product of glucose, fat, or protein metabolism can enter a "feeder pathway" that we know as the Krebs cycle (another popular science phrase that's fun to cavalierly insert into conversations without the expectation of any legitimate understanding of its enzymes, intermediates, or purpose). This process occurs in the MITOCHONDRIAL MATRIX. So the Krebs cycle spins and produces a little energy (adenosine triphosphate, or ATP) as well as some charitable electron donors which enter the ELECTRON TRANSPORT CHAIN. This is where all this electrical energy can be converted to chemical energy. Normally, the electrons are smoothly transferred from each complex of the electron transport chain, and you can think of this as if your "cellular battery" is getting fully charged up. HOWEVER, if you're insulin resistant or hyperglycemic or both, reactive oxygen species (ROS) are generated instead of ATP. You're basically leaking battery acid all over your cells, which is no good. Exercise, for many reasons, enables you to better charge up your cellular batteries rather than inefficiently seeping free radicals...and we all know how embarrassing seepage can be.

b. Heavy weights won't pick themselves up, and no one ever said, "I wish that I was weaker." Lift some weights. Compound movements such as squats, deadlift variations, pressing, vertical pulls, and horizontal pulls utilizing large muscle groups will give you the most bang for your buck (obviously within the parameters of your orthopedic limitations). Doing tricep kickbacks with pink weights doesn't count.
   i. Remember that access code to your cellular suitcases, GLUT4? Well GLUT4 is an INSULIN-DEPENDENT transporter and is how glucose gets into your INSULIN-DEPENDENT tissues, which are your MUSCLE and your FAT cells. But what's awesome about exercise is that it allows you complimentary cellular access WITHOUT needing INSULIN... yes, you can get glucose INTO YOUR CELLS WITHOUT INSULIN! The exercise itself leads to GLUT4 translocation to the cell surface and subsequent glucose uptake for utilization. Basically, you're like that gym bro who gets an honorary lifetime GLUT4 cellular membership without paying the hormonal price when you exercise...pretty awesome and pretty important, especially since the first place that insulin resistance starts is skeletal muscle.

c. Training for power is of critical importance as you age; your fast-twitch Type II muscle fibers tend to shift toward slow-twitch Type I fibers over time. And if you want to be able to chase your grandkids across the playground, incorporating some form of speedwork/plyometric work into your regimen is underrated and underappreciated. Many people never sprint again after they turn 30...that's pretty

sad, especially since running fast is awesome. (If you haven't sprinted for the last 15 years, don't go crazy...I don't want you tearing your hamstring or Achilles or both...there's a proper way to get back into the groove). But the best strategy is just don't ever stop.

4. Lather, rinse, repeat. Consistency is key. The people who are the most metabolically healthy are the ones who started moving when they were young and never stopped.

I know that within my framework the maintenance of normal blood glucose parameters is only Pillar 1 of the Home Security System. A complete lack of insulin is incompatible with life, but most chronic disease is driven in large part by too much insulin. Ergo, almost everything falls into place if you take the appropriate measures to "Control your insulin, control your life."

DEEP DIVE: Anti-diabetic Drugs

Sulfonylureas

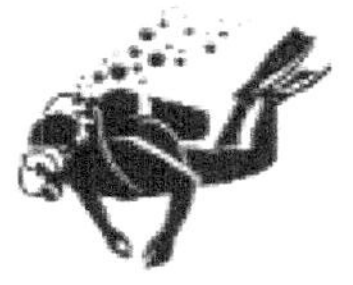

If you want to make your patient fatter, induce hypoglycemia, burn out his or her pancreas, and likely increase the risk of heart attacks and strokes, by all means prescribe a sulfonylurea. "But sulfonylureas are cheap!" Yeah, you know what else is inexpensive? Fasting. Outside of some rare MODY variants that result in "Type 1.5" diabetes, sulfonylureas are basically malpractice.

There's another class of medications called meglitinides that are basically sulfonylureas, but these drugs at least have the decency to wait until blood sugars are actually elevated to make you make insulin; this results in a few less hypoglycemic episodes. So if clinicians merely dislike their patients rather than abjectly despising them, perhaps they would prescribe a meglitinide.

Thiazolidenediones

Mercifully, we will heretofore refer to this class as TZDs, and the only medication available is Pioglitazone. Pioglitazone basically makes you fatter in a less malignant way; it redistributes fat from visceral depots to subcutaneous reserves. So you get a little chunkier, but everything else gets better. It's a potent vasodilator, which is why it's contraindicated in heart failure due to increasing edema (although it may actually improve ejection fraction in that population...interesting stuff).

So should you "Get in the Zone with Pioglitazone?" Well, maybe. In my experience, populations from Southeast Asia with normal BMIs but terrible diabetes benefit immensely from Pioglitazone. It makes them fatter in a better way, reducing the highly inflammatory visceral fat that plagues this population who has a genetically low "liposusceptibility threshold." Pioglitazone often unfairly gets thrown into the same undignified bucket as sulfonylureas, since it was a "First Generation" medication, but definitely keep Pioglitazone available in your toolbox.

Metformin

France has contributed many luminaries to science, including Pascal and Descartes, but maybe Metformin deserves a place on this proverbial intellectual *Mont Blanc* as well. Derived from the French lilac, Metformin continues to be a source of controversy and diarrhea for both scientists and patients across the world. Smart people like to debate whether or not its inhibition of the electron transport chain really occurs at clinical doses, while others pontificate over the mechanism by which it modulates the nutrient sensor AMPK. And anyone who has ever taken big doses of Metformin knows that it can almost make a colonoscopy bowel prep seem tame.

I really don't care too much, but what I'll say is that Metformin seems to blunt some of the beneficial effects of exercise, so although it's not a useless tool by any means, it's not my favorite. But if Metformin is the catalyst to get people who haven't run in a decade running to the bathroom, then maybe that's a good thing. At least it's not a sulfonylurea.

Acarbose

Sometimes, the best part about medicine is it provides ample fodder for jocularity. And that's really the main reason why Acarbose exists. Acarbose is an alpha-glucosidase inhibitor; or a "starch-blocker" in plain language. Essentially, if you take it on "Cheat Day" prior to binging on endless breadsticks at Olive Garden, it attenuates the spike in blood sugars that would otherwise result.

However, if you're going to employ this approach, you better make sure you're in the presence of those who unconditionally love you. Because the flatulence that inevitably ensues can only be described as volcanic.

So is Acarbose useless? Nope, and I did use it on several occasions in lieu of prandial insulin for some rather non-compliant individuals...their CGMs suggested that was a reasonable intervention. But was it worth acquiring the nickname "Fart Simpson" in the process?" You'll have to ask them...if you can stand to be in the same room.

SGLT2 Inhibitors

Ralph DeFronzo is like the Chuck Norris of physicians; medical board exams aspire to get certified in DeFronzo rather than the other way around. Even the collateral debris from the knowledge bombs he drops on a minute-by-minute basis generally end up being priceless gems for us mere mortals.

DeFronzo's piquant answer to the question, "What goes wrong in Type 2 diabetes?" is famously described as the Ominous Octet. And one of those core defects is excessive glucose reabsorption at the proximal convoluted tubule of the kidney via a transporter called SGLT2. Basically, in the catastrophic confusion of hyperglycemia, your body thinks it needs even MORE sugar even though your body is literally saturated with it. So by inhibiting this sodium-glucose co-transporter, you end up peeing out the excess sugar rather than reabsorbing it. People were concerned that peeing out all that sugar would damage the kidneys, but DeFronzo, as usual, was correct that this mechanism would actually prove beneficial for not only lowering blood sugar, but also protecting the kidneys. It just comes with an increased risk of yeast infections, since you become a purveyor of Sweet Pee.

And this class of medication, which is anything that ends in -flozin, has a broad range of benefits to help people "Get Back in the Flo." They have shown benefit in reducing heart failure complications, high uric acid, proteinuria, and even epicardial fat. SGLT2 inhibitors actually help your myocardium, which has become terrible at using other fuel sources, utilize ketones to help minimize "fatty heart." Basically, if someone has diabetes, hyperuricemia, atrial fibrillation, chronic kidney disease or proteinuria, these medications will probably have some benefit in restoring the integrity of the Home Security System.

GLP-1 Receptor Agonists and Incretin Mimetics (basically most things that end in Tide)

The last class of medications we will discuss is not only a pharmaceutical, but a cultural phenomenon. When asked the question, "What do incretin mimetics, including GLP-1 receptor agonists, do for you?," the answer is "Pretty much everything." They have proven benefit in reducing a host of cardiovascular events as well as the number on your bathroom scale, and they may even have some benefit in neurodegenerative disease.

So what are incretins? These are gut peptides, including GIP and GLP-1, that help augment the postprandial insulin response to ingested nutrients. Under normal physiologic conditions, incretins account for 2/3 of the appropriate insulin response to eating, with GIP actually the majority player. However, when everything goes wrong (diabesity), this incretin effect is lost, so incretin modulators at supraphysiologic concentrations may be required to restore normalcy.

These drugs, as stated, potentially affect almost every organ system, but really they restore your body's ability to use its Savings Account when it comes to fuel partitioning. And they potently do this, in large part, by reducing appetite. Oftentimes folks with insulin resistance are plagued by perpetual "food noise," and these medications organize the orchestra so you can symphonically "Control your insulin, control your life."

Whenever I go fill up my car with gas, I don't call up my friends and post about it on Social Media to encourage all of them to join me at Chevron Pump #4. I just fuel up and then carry on with my life. Similarly, these medications help shift people's mindset regarding food to one of "fueling the machine," rather than mealtimes being the most significant hedonic events of the day. They really do help catalyze a dietary shift from the Standard American Disaster to one that prioritizes protein and eats real food.

So what are the downsides to these miracle drugs? Well, if you insist on indulging in tater tots and nachos while on a GLP-1RA, you'll puke your guts out, which is sort of the point. And if you're a rat with Multiple Endocrine Neoplasia Type 2, then by all means stay away. But the major concern with these medications is the loss of MUSCLE MASS; you don't want to be trading one problem (obesity) for another (sarcopenia). And the amount of lean mass loss observed in clinical trials is certainly significant.

But can this problem be avoided? Absolutely, but it requires RESISTANCE EXERCISE along with adequate dietary protein, specifically protein containing sufficient quantities of the amino acid leucine. There are 2 main stimuli for mTORC1 in skeletal muscle, which is the anabolic (growth) switch that you WANT turned on in muscle. The most important is the imposed stressor of the resistance exercise itself, and the second is sufficient leucine, so if you ensure that these issues are being addressed, you ought to be ok.

You may very well skip lunch while taking semaglutide, but there's no proverbial "free lunch" when it comes to attenuating the otherwise inevitable decrease in muscle mass while on an incretin-based therapy. Go pick up some heavy things. And when you do eat, maybe swap out the cheese puffs for some cottage cheese.

Dipeptidyl Peptidase-4 Inhibitors

There's an enzyme called DPP-4 that degrades both GIP and GLP-1, so inhibiting that enzyme to theoretically increase the availability of circulating incretins seemed like a reasonable strategy at one point. And drugs ending in -gliptin came to market employing this mechanistic approach...with rather underwhelming results. They lowered blood sugars a little, but didn't meaningfully reduce cardiovascular events...and then the GLP-1 receptor agonists came along and pretty much rendered this class obsolete.

Using a gliptin in the Age of Ozempic is like selecting Chris Rock to play Thor when Chris Hemsworth is available. One is clearly better suited for the role than the other...although there would probably be a few more laughs if clinicians insisted on using Januvia over Mounjaro.

PILLAR 2: KEEP BLOOD PRESSURE NORMAL

"I almost hit a squirrel driving over here, so I'm sure that's the reason."
"Well, you know it's that "white coat syndrome" kicking in..."
"My bottom number is good and that's the most important one."
-Common patient excuses justifying the "normalcy" of their systolic blood pressure of 190

Systolic blood pressure is the pressure exerted in your arteries when your heart beats (ventricular contraction), which is 1/3 of your cardiac cycle. And diastolic blood pressure is the force on your arteries during the remaining 2/3 of the cardiac cycle when your heart chambers are refilling and preparing to do it all over again. Both are important, although the bulk of research suggests the "bottom number" isn't quite as important as the "top number" when it comes to risk of cardiovascular events. Regardless, the association of elevated blood pressure with cardiovascular events is well-documented, and various trials such as SPRINT and more recently BPROAD show that lower blood pressure reduces the incidence of cardiovascular events over time. People don't say, "Wow, I feel like my blood pressure is sky-high," when life is full of stress-free whimsy, puppies, and ice cream (or Chobani Zero Greek yogurt if you open my refrigerator). Contents under pressure are liable to explode, and the litany of physiologic regulators that maintain blood pressure in a tightly controlled range speaks to its importance. For example:

- Short-term regulation of BP is dictated by BARORECEPTORS. These sense rapid changes in PRESSURE (think that if you're being chased by a bear-o, there's a lot of pressure on you to get away-o). And this is the rapid equilibration that occurs when you've been lying down and then you stand up...sometimes there is a sluggish response and you feel a little woozy, and we call this orthostatic hypotension. But typically you figure it out pretty quick since it's not in your best interest to pass out.
- Long-term regulation of BP is HORMONALLY mediated, and since BP is so important, a whole bunch of organs get involved; it's a beautiful example of physiologic teamwork in action primarily orchestrated by the RAAS (renin-angiotensin-aldosterone system).
    - The **kidney** initially senses less pressure coming into it via one of its "little arteries" called the afferent arteriole and secretes a protein called **renin.**
    - Meanwhile, the liver creates a precursor called **angiotensinogen.** (Whenever you see the suffix -gen in biology it generally means it's an inactive precursor that needs some sort of enzymatic help to generate the active product). And **renin** is the guy who makes **angiotensin 1** from its precursor.
    - Then, the **lungs** see all the excitement and, not wanting to miss out on some critical homeostatic regulation, uses the enzyme angiotensin converting enzyme, or **ACE** (which you've probably heard of in reference to ACE inhibitors like Lisinopril) to

convert **angiotensin 1** to **angiotensin 2**. The little guy that started as an inactive precursor has now mature!
  - Just when you think that no more organs could possibly join the party, the **adrenal glands** get the message from **angiotensin 2** to generate the steroid hormone **aldosterne.**
  - Finally, **aldosterone** has a variety of effects on different organs including the kidney, blood vessels, and heart, acting as a **vasoconstrictor**...and anytime the pipes get narrower, BP incrases.
- There are other regulators such as antidiuretic hormone, various natriuretic peptides, and chemoreceptors, but I guess the main point here is that YOUR BODY HAS PRIORITIZED BLOOD PRESSURE REGULATION. So you should too.

So let's say your BP is elevated, and I'm going to take the liberty of eliminating the squirrel and "white coat syndrome" as the possible causes. Here's a short list of questions you probably SHOULDN'T first ask yourself if you're a little on the hypertensive side:

1. Do I need to get an abdominal CT scan to see if I have some sort of adrenal tumor?
2. Did my thyroid or parathyroid glands go berserk?
3. Do I have something structurally wrong with my kidney?
4. Have I inadvertently been eating obscene amounts of licorice? (Seriously though, there's something called glycyrrhizin in licorice that legitimately can elevate your BP. Also, licorice is gross).

Now, all those rare secondary causes (and many more) are possible, but there would likely be other symptoms that would cause you to embark on a proverbial zebra-hunting diagnostic safari. Instead, some questions that you SHOULD ask yourself if you're having high BP would be these:

1. **Do I have some extra weight to lose?**
   a. If so, you're probably insulin resistant...take the necessary measures to "control your insulin, control your life."
2. **Am I truly in "fighting shape" in regards to body composition? Am I aggressively (or even modestly) pulling the exercise lever?**
   a. If not, you're probably insulin resistant...take the necessary measures to "control your insulin, control your life."
3. **Do I have sleep apnea? Did we recently have to buy a new house just so my spouse could have his or her own bedroom?**
   a. If so, ask yourself Questions 1 and 2. If the answer is Yes to Question 1 and/or No to Question 2, most sleep apnea is directly impacted by insulin resistance...so take the necessary measures to "control your insulin, control your life."

And then, if you rectify your metabolic health and you're feeling much more like the Spartan you were in your 20's, your BP has probably normalized and you're back to absolutely crushing it at life. BUT, there are a few other related factors to consider that can not only jeopardize your blood pressure, but compromise your Home Security System as a whole. And that's what brings us to the next series of important questions:

1. **Am I drinking too much fructose?**
   a. Soda and fruit juices are the real offenders here, and fructose is metabolized in a unique manner, actually

resulting in a transient depletion in intracellular energy. So there is zero satiety signal, zero feedback inhibition, and before you know it, your confused cells think they're starving when they're really getting saturated in a sugary cesspool. And fructose turns on genes that result in LIPOGENESIS (fat production) and also produces URIC ACID.

i. Uric acid is well known for causing gout, and this happens because at high concentrations it crystallizes once in the extracellular space. Classically, this results in a painful and swollen big toe, but it can occur in other joints as well. However, it also wreaks havoc INSIDE the cell. Remember your savings account and how we should be using fat as fuel? Well, the second enzymatic step in breaking down fat to use as fuel (called enoyl-CoA hydratase) is actually INHIBITED by uric acid. And remember the mitochondrial powerhouse? Well, one of the enzymes that keeps the Krebs cycle spinning is called aconitase...and uric acid INHIBITS aconitase as well. Oh yeah, and remember that eNOS that functions as a potent vasodilator? Well, uric acid INHIBITS that, too, resulting in elevated blood pressure. No wonder elevated uric acid is associated with increased progression of coronary plaque as well as cardiovascular mortality.

2. **Am I drinking too much alcohol?**
    a. And just like that, the lighthearted conviviality screeches to a halt as a deafening silence encapsulates the room...but trust me, we'll make this fun.

So, a few disclaimers before we embark on a somewhat tangential, but ultimately worthwhile exploration of this elixir:

1. Obviously if you're an adult of legal drinking age, it's absolutely fine to enjoy alcoholic beverages responsibly.
2. I personally don't drink, but not primarily for biochemical reasons. I have the privilege of doing the Youth Ministries at my church, and since the Common Sense and Context cortices are, at best, underdeveloped in this demographic, I feel it's best for me to not ever drink at all in order to maximize my influence on them as someone to whom they look to as a mentor.
3. I always think it's funny that if you have elected to abstain from ethanol, you are obligated to explain yourself. Can you imagine if you had to justify your rationale for mayonnaise avoidance? "My grandfather's life was ruined by mayonnaise, so I just think it's best that I never start down that road..."
4. Although, as you'll see, I believe the optimal amount of alcohol consumption for metabolic health to be zero, if you hold a contrarian view you can always cherry-pick through the literature to find a study or two that will justify your position.
   a. On a somewhat related note, one of my personal favorite cherry-picking ventures involves a study suggesting that people with larger brains tend to take more naps. Naps are absolutely delicious, so if I ever doze off around 3 PM I attribute this to the physiologic requirement necessary to optimize my brain volume.

Ok, here are the physiologic results of alcohol consumption. Feel free to skip to the next chapter if this is a trigger.

1. Like fructose, alcohol increases uric acid (see above), inhibits eNOS, and elevates blood pressure. Remember, optimizing blood pressure is actually the topic of this chapter.
2. Alcohol disrupts the normal ratios in both the cytoplasm and mitochondrial compartments of the cell of something called NAD+ and NADH (these are the oxidized and reduced forms of nicotinamide adenine dinucleotide...don't worry about it). Normally, there is relatively more NAD+ compared to NADH, and the continuation of normal processes such as the Krebs cycle and gluconeogenesis depend on optimizing these cellular ratios. However, since NADH is a byproduct of alcohol metabolism, the Krebs cycle screeches to a halt, and it simultaneously impairs your body's ability to generate its own glucose supply. However, NADH also turns on lipogenic enzymes...it's a hot mess in which you can literally have HYPOGLYCEMIA (low blood sugars), enter a state of METABOLIC ACIDOSIS, and get fatter all at the same time. Your body pretty much short circuits.
3. One of the byproducts of alcohol metabolism, acetaldehyde, is a carcinogen, and alcohol is associated with multiple cancers, including liver and breast cancer.
4. Speaking of breasts, for you gentlemen alcohol can reduce your testosterone and increase your estrogen. This can result in gynecomastia, or more colloquially "moobs." Not generally a great life goal.
5. Alcohol can increase your cortisol (stress hormone), interferes with normal sleep cycles (despite it being a CNS depressant), and no one includes alcohol in their favorite Brain Clarity cocktail for obvious reasons.
6. Alcohol increases your risk of atrial fibrillation, which increases your risk of having a stroke, and long-term can

result in dilated cardiomyopathy (you've got a big heart...it just doesn't work).

7. It's a neurotoxin, liver toxin, and toxic to your mitochondria.
8. Other than that, it's pretty healthy.

But wait, you say...doesn't it increase my "good cholesterol," the HDL? Yep, but as you'll see in a few chapters, HDL is capable of doing some good things, but as a biomarker tells you NOTHING about the functionality of that particle. And high HDL doesn't necessarily protect you from heart disease, particularly if it's high from alcohol use. Sorry.

How to Measure Your Blood Pressure

Slap on a cuff and check it.

Ok, so let's say you want to get a little more granular and this discussion about alcohol has made you thirsty for sophistication and nuance. Is there a test or combination of tests that can give you a better indication of your endothelial function? Sure, you could go deep down the rabbit hole and get a brachial FMD, measure something called asymmetric/symmetric dimethylarginine (ADMA/SDMA), find a lab to test your F2 isoprostanes and malondialdehyde, and then go hunt for the 7 or 8 people on the planet that might be able to help you make sense of all that stuff. You could check uric acid, which is a little more pragmatic (and actionable...there are even a few medications such as SGLT2 inhibitors and some xanthine oxidase inhibitors that reduce uric acid, which might be helpful occasionally). But I'd say that perhaps the best, cheapest, most practical test in addition to just simply taking your blood pressure would be a test for urinary microalbumin, often called a UACR. Basically, you pee and see if there's protein in your pee, which shouldn't ever be there. (Pea protein is also terrible, both in taste and ability to provide adequate amino acid requirements for muscle protein synthesis). It's pretty much the standard to check UACR in people with diabetes...but even in people without diabetes or hypertension in the EPIC-NORFOLK study, elevated urinary microalbumin was associated with a 148% increased risk of all-cause mortality and a 203% increase of dying from cardiovascular disease. If you are leaking protein in your urine, your Home Security System is not as robust as you think, and it tells you that prompt action is necessary to repair your compromised physiologic dwelling.

PILLAR 3: KEEP INFLAMMATION LOW

"There is a strength of conviction that can only come from being 100% wrong."
-Stephen Schneider

Social media influencers make their livings on a smorgasbord of logical fallacies, aesthetic manipulation, the appeal of novelty, iconoclastic rhetoric, and captivatingly charismatic oratory. If it looks good and sounds good, you can easily prey on the human behavioral tendency to be sheep-like, particularly when the status quo is suboptimal. For instance, with absolute conviction, someone can declare that "inadequate methylation is the true source of all your thyroid problems," and that if you get some super expensive genetic testing, you can identify the "root cause," rectify your existential angst, and possess boundless energy typically only seen in those on amphetamines. Does it matter that the thyroid gland has nothing to do with methylation (a methyl group is a carbon atom with 3 hydrogens attached) and that actual conversion of thyroxine (T4) to active T3 actually requires deiodination (removal of an iodine from the parent molecule)? Nope! Because you're chronically tired and the person articulating this message of hope seems reasonably healthy and remarkably self-assured. And maybe, just maybe, if you were better at recycling homocysteine to methionine you, too, could have his same level of exuberance and confidence!

In my Sophomore Honors English class (that seems to be a pivotal year for me), we were doing a module on free verse poetry. And a few of the poems were ok, but most of them were either esoteric, unintelligible, or just plain infantile...one guy would completely defenestrate proper punctuation and it was hailed as "creative genius" and another would commit grammatical suicide and be labeled as a "pioneer." And so I thought, "I'm going to write my own free verse poem." So as I was sitting in Microbiology class, I looked around the room and wrote down a hodgepodge of random, inchoate associations combined with vague references to some of the events I had just learned about in World History. Did it have any real meaning? Absolutely not. But somehow, despite its ludicrous content, it retained an aura of provocative poignancy that a reader could possibly misinterpret as possessing "deeper significance." I titled it, "*The Tapestry,*" and volunteered to read it in front of my class. I was completely transparent in explaining my satirical intent, and shockingly, my teacher was not amused. I pretended to be offended, and said, "Well fine...I'm going to submit it to the National Poetry contest." AND IT WON. Not the grand prize, but it was a regional winner and ended up being published in some anthology. I felt righteously vindicated, but more so just amused at the image of some pseudo-intellectual in a Starbucks somewhere trying to offer a fresh critique of *The Tapestry's* mysterious message.

Everyone seems to have a fresh take on "inflammation," and if you ask 10 people to define inflammation, you'll probably get 10 different answers. And millions of dollars are spent each year in a quest to be "less inflamed." Who do you believe? Who can we trust? These are difficult questions, which is why I try to root my rationales in the physiology and biochemistry that the good Lord Himself created. Otherwise, you might be persuaded to think that the proprietary blend of various shrubbery fragments and B vitamins will fix your inflammation...or that *The Tapestry* is actually a piece of classic literature.

So is inflammation inherently bad? Well, without a proper inflammatory response, every little virus or bacterium could kill you off pretty quick, and there is a militia of cytokines, interleukins, macrophages, various white blood cell types, and other chemical mediators that ideally work together to neutralize foreign invaders. With inflammation, just like many other topics in medicine, CONTEXT MATTERS. We all want these inflammatory markers and players to be a binary discussion; good or bad, protective or disastrous, but it's rarely that simple.

A good example of this is my favorite interleukin, interleukin-6 (IL-6). Yes, I have a favorite interleukin, which at this point is probably not super surprising. Although not widely tested, IL-6 as a biomarker is associated with cardiovascular disease and people with certain genetic variants in the *IL6* gene also have increased risk for cardiac events. But IL-6 has PRO-INFLAMMATORY or ANTI-INFLAMMATORY functions depending on its ORIGIN and depending on the CONTEXT. If it's secreted as an adipokine from a fat cell, it leads to chronic low-grade systemic inflammation. BUT, if it's released in a large quantity all at once from skeletal muscle in response to exercise, then it has ANTI-INFLAMMATORY effects. Same interleukin, different origin story, different results. Context matters!

Another example of this tricky topic is a tribe of hunter-gatherers called the Tsimane in Bolivia. These people, on average, have a high-sensitivity C-reactive protein (hs-CRP) of 9.2 mg/L! HS-CRP is a commercially available, widely used biomarker of non-specific inflammation. Normally you should be below 1, between 1 and 2 is getting a little sketchy, and anything over 2 is elevated...and high hs-CRP is an INDEPENDENT RISK FACTOR for cardiovascular disease. And their IL-6 levels are high as well...so these people must have raging heart disease, right? Wrong! That population is virtually free from cardiovascular events...the reason these inflammatory markers are high is that the Tsimane are riddled with parasites, and these various inflammatory mediators are merely fighting off nasty critters. Context matters!

Once you've identified markers of inflammation, addressing the ROOT CAUSE of that inflammation is more important than just getting rid of every cytokine or interleukin or protein that might be making you inflamed. We don't all just proactively take Advil to mitigate our risk of heart attacks. Now don't get me wrong, elevated inflammation is certainly an independent factor in regards to risk of heart disease, and several studies such as CANTOS and a couple of colchicine trials demonstrated reduction in cardiovascular events by neutralizing the inflammatory component. But other trials using anti-inflammatory agents like methotrexate didn't work, and another more recent colchicine trial failed as well.

If C5 ain't MAC-ing, it could be PLAQUE-ing!

The complement cascade is an important part of the innate immune response and involves a bunch of proteins that form the Membrane Attack Complex, or MAC. Plasma levels of one these proteins, C5, is actually associated with a 30-50% greater likelihood of having multivessel disease in several cohorts, including PESA. So, once again, the maladaptive immune response in the context of "mailmen going rogue" can be problematic! If C5 ain't MAC-ing, it could be PLAQUE-ing!

As stated, hs-CRP is widely available and although other markers such as the aforementioned IL-6 and something called

GlycA may have potentially more utility in the future, CRP is a reasonable blood test to obtain at this time. And if it's elevated, we can then ask some specific questions to help better elucidate the root cause of this anomaly:

1. **Do I have some extra weight to lose? Am I truly at my "fighting weight" in regards to body composition?** (These questions should look familiar).
   a. Most elevations in hs-CRP are due to ANGRY FAT. Remember the macrophages that tend to be M1 proinflammatory guys when you're insulin resistant? And remember the IL-6 that is pro-inflammatory when released from fat cells? (IL-6 is one of the many things that tells your liver to make CRP). When adjusted for waist circumference and total fat mass, CRP mostly (not all the way), but mostly goes away as a meaningful marker.
2. **Do I have a systemic autoimmune disease?**
   a. Certain conditions such as psoriasis, lupus, and rheumatoid arthritis are associated with chronic systemic inflammation and increased risk of cardiovascular disease. It's an unfortunate hand to be dealt, but hopefully you can corral a great group of health care professionals to help you navigate this case of "picking the wrong parents." Thankfully, these things aren't incredibly common and can be managed. And addressing the aspects of your Home Security System that you *can* control always helps!
3. **Do I have right lower quadrant pain and a super high fever?**
   a. You have appendicitis, so go get an appendectomy and your CRP will come down.

Inflammation certainly matters. But most of the time in America, instead of neutralizing parasites, your inflammatory team resents your state of overnutrition and gets back at you by attacking your vascular endothelium. Control your insulin, control your life, and your interleukins and cytokines will usually fall in line.

PILLAR 4: SMOKING AND DRUGS

Coach Limbago was a legend at Meridian Elementary. He possessed a magnetic *je ne sais quais*, and our cohort of perpetually disheveled and generally unfocused rapscallions actually hung on his every word. When he taught us how to count to ten in Hawaiian, we learned. When he ordered us to do push-ups, we immediately dropped down to our bellies to see whose spaghetti arms could churn out the most repetitions. We all wanted to make Coach proud, and the telltale sign of his approval was a flaring of his nostrils accompanied by a twinkle of his caramel eyes. I elicited this response from Coach every time I nailed a hapless opponent during dodgeball with ruthless and precocious velocity, so I was convinced he had a special affection for me.

And every year during Red Ribbon Week, Coach would bring his ukulele to school and play the "Drug Free" song. It went something like this:

Everybody knows I'm a happy kid
I don't do drugs, smoke, drink or fib
I'm the happiest kid you'll ever see
And I choose to stay DRUG FREE!

This last line was repeated with increasing volume and gusto somewhere between three and 300 times. And so with fists thrust heavenward, 800 unruly scalawags at Meridian Elementary committed to never, ever even entertaining the notion of abusing illicit substances. Coach said so...that was good enough for me.

Well, Coach eventually retired, but apparently they still participate in Red Ribbon Week at the local schools. The reason I know this is because I saw a group of kids wearing those timeless Red Ribbons a few weeks ago...but upon further inspection, two of them were vaping. This generation needs Coach and his ukulele more than ever.

So please, remember what Coach taught us when it comes to smoking and drugs. Despite what the kids may be doing, the rules actually haven't changed.

Don't. Just don't.

PART II

THE LIPID NEIGHBORHOOD

1

ENTERING THE LIPID NEIGHBORHOOD

"LDL bad, HDL good, everyone take a statin."
-Pretty much every medical program when it comes to cholesterol and lipid education

I first recognized mediocrity's insidious and pervasive societal effects when I was in first grade. Underneath my hideous blonde bowl-cut was an eager and focused mind; my parents had told me to "do my best in school" and I took that commitment very seriously. Additionally, I loved learning, and after I would finish my regular classwork, I would do what any normal kid would do; I would see if I could memorize all the statistics on my baseball cards as well as the capitals of every nation on the planet. (I still remember all those capitals, but whenever I suggest playing the game "African Nations and their Capitals," at family get-togethers, people always seem to "need to leave early"). But anyway, after about a month of school, my teacher announced that I had received an award for my scholastic performance. This award involved a certificate, a cinnamon roll, and having my picture taken with the principal at the "Breakfast of Champions" ceremony. I was on cloud nine, and I proudly used 4 magnets to secure my certificate on the refrigerator so it wouldn't fall down.

As the school year went on, other students received invitations to additional "Breakfast of Champions" ceremonies. It made sense that Caleb Bastian received the award, since he was actually literate, and I didn't have too much of an issue when Jessica Tanford was similarly honored. But as the year progressed, every single one of my classmates gradually ended up being a "Champion," and the last straw was when Michael Weatherby received the award. Michael's right index finger was perpetually macerated from being in his nose and he spent most of his time in the office because of his insistence on being a Champion of Delinquency. And the day I heard that Michael had "achieved" this award, I went home after school and tore my certificate off the refrigerator. And ever since then, I have been on a personal crusade against mediocrity, which unfortunately has seeped deeply into the fabric of the medical establishment.

And I get it, lipids are HARD. Take a look at this picture, which merely scratches the surface of the complexities of cholesterol homeostasis:

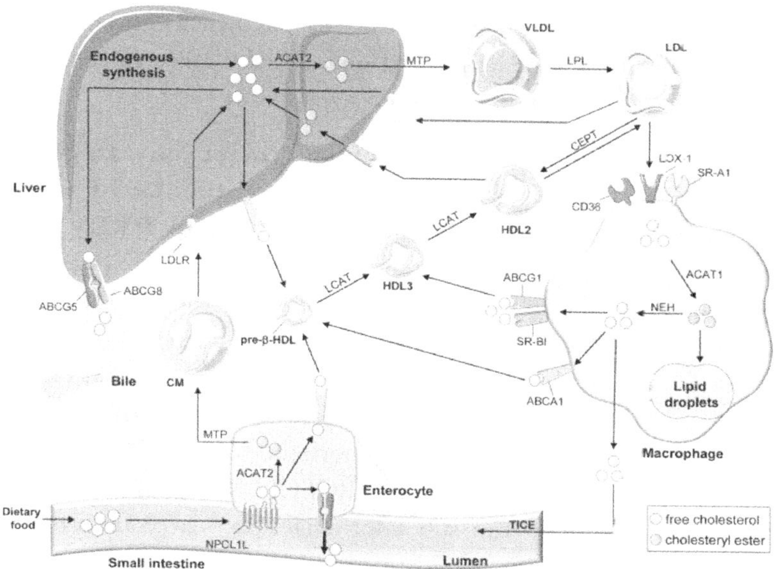

Figure 3: "Lipid Transport...it's really quite simple." Source: Duan, Y., Gong, K., Xu, S., Zhang, F., Meng, X., & Han, J. (2022). Regulation of cholesterol homeostasis in health and diseases: from mechanisms to targeted therapeutics. *Signal transduction and targeted therapy*, *7*(1), 265. https://doi.org/10.1038/s41392-022-01125-5

I precepted medical students, PA students, and NP students, and it's true that most of the time all they were ever taught about lipids was "LDL bad, HDL good, everyone take a statin." And if we were discussing some orphan disease that affects a couple people every now and then, maybe that would be acceptable. But these lipid mediators are critical players in the NUMBER ONE KILLER OF PEOPLE ACROSS THE WORLD, and I believe one of the biggest reasons we haven't made meaningful progress in treating cardiovascular disease is that we continue to foster a culture of mediocrity rather than transcendence. Additionally, this leads to a trickle-down effect once students become practitioners. Primary care providers assume that "the cardiologist will take care of it." And maybe the cardiologist will...or not. And maybe the cardiologist assumes that the Endocrinologist or Lipid Specialist will manage the cholesterol metrics. But maybe the patient never shows up for the appointment...and maybe no one actually takes care of the problem. If everyone punts, no one ever scores!

So whether you're a clinician or not, my goal for you is **to NOT have heart attacks, strokes, and dementia. And I want to shift the paradigm from REACTION to PREVENTION**. We know how important the Home Security System is, but this next section will further elaborate on the Lipid Neighborhood in which every ApoB-containing particle, the vast majority typically being LDL, is potentially a criminal that could infiltrate your physiologic home. And maybe you have some of those Lp(a) "felons" in your neighborhood as well. But regardless, you CANNOT HAVE ATHEROSCLEROSIS without one of these particles in the subendothelial space of your arterial wall. And that's why we need to understand your Lipid Neighborhood.

As we explore the Lipid Neighborhood, it's going to get a little wild at times, so ground yourself in these 5 core concepts:

1. **A lack of cholesterol is incompatible with life.**
2. **There is a big difference between PLASMA cholesterol and CELLULAR cholesterol**...if you had any cellular deficiency in cholesterol, you wouldn't be alive, let alone reading this book. And what you see on your cholesterol blood panel, which is the amount in plasma, is only about 10% of your total body cholesterol.
3. Blood is mostly water, and fat and water don't mix, **so we need LIPOPROTEINS as the vehicles to transport LIPIDS.**
4. **The purpose of these LIPOPROTEINS is NOT to give you heart disease. Lipoproteins are simply MAILMEN.** Most mailmen aren't bad dudes. Their job is to deliver the mail (triglycerides primarily) and then go home (to the liver) at the end of the day.

However, if that mailman runs his truck into your arterial wall, that's a bad mailman and we need to do something about it.

5. **Once again, you CANNOT have atherosclerosis without one of these mailmen going rogue and running his truck into your arterial wall**. It's at the scene of this crime that a maladaptive immune response ensues, resulting in plaque formation, which can ultimately lead to a cardiovascular event.

2

WHAT IS CHOLESTEROL?

Perhaps no organic molecule has been subject to as much unjustified demonization as *cholesterol.* A lack of cholesterol is incompatible with life. Cholesterol serves a critical role in the following:

- Cholesterol is an essential structural component in cell membranes.
- It functions as a precursor to steroid hormones, including cortisol, aldosterone, testosterone, estrogens, and vitamin D.
- Bile acids are formed from cholesterol and are essential in maintaining normal digestive function.
- 20-25% of total body cholesterol is in the brain, and cholesterol serves a critical role in a variety of important processes in the central nervous system (more on that later).
- Cholesterol, along with other lipid friends, are indispensable components of the skin epidermal layer.

Given its ubiquity and importance, it's no wonder that **every nucleated cell in your body is capable of synthesizing**

cholesterol. And the amount of cholesterol in the cell is very tightly regulated. Cellular deficiency is incompatible with life, but cellular excess of cholesterol is toxic and leads to the cell "committing suicide" in a process called *apoptosis*. Excess cholesterol can also form crystals (kind of like uric acid in gout) and this can consequently make coronary plaques more vulnerable to rupture.

So there's a sweet spot, and already the terms "good cholesterol" and "bad cholesterol" should strike you as silly...the same 27-carbon, 4-ringed aromatic molecule is the same regardless of where it's located...it's just a matter of whether it's ESTERIFIED or UNESTERIFIED, which will be explained below.

So let's take a look at the structure of cholesterol in **Figure 4:**

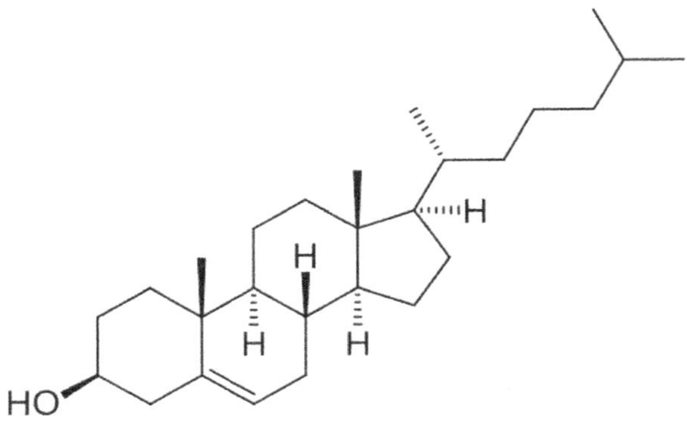

If you look at this picture, this would be "FREE CHOLESTEROL." Off of the 3rd carbon in the first ring, you'll see an -OH, and then you can exclaim, "Oh look, it's a hydroxyl group!" (I never know which of my silly mnemonics might stick with you, so I'll use them all). In order for cholesterol to be processed into a steroid hormone or form a bile acid or function in a cell membrane, it has to be in this "free and unburdened"

form. But most of your body's cholesterol, at least below the brain, is in its storage, or ESTERIFIED form. If we substitute a FATTY ACID for the HYDROXYL group, then it is ESTERIFIED and subsequently referred to as a CHOLESTERYL ESTER. This is super lame, but I ask my students the question, "Why is **Esther** so **fat**?" and this sometimes helps them remember the fatty acid attachment that esterifies the molecule along with the proper nomenclature. (If your name is Esther, please don't be offended...I'm sure you're a metabolic powerhouse who "Controls her insulin, controls her life."

So to recap:

- ESTERIFIED cholesterol is its storage form.
- For cholesterol to be utilized for steroidogenesis or whatever else, it must be DE-ESTERIFIED.

You'll also notice that most of the bonds in this structure are single, saturated bonds, but there is a conspicuous double bond between carbons 5 and 6 in the 2nd ring. If you reduce that bond (make it a single bond), then the molecule becomes CHOLESTANOL, which can't serve any purpose in the body except proceed into the toilet bowl when you go Number 2. Cholestanol really shouldn't ever be reabsorbed into your body to any appreciable degree.

Cholesterol Synthesis

The process of cholesterol synthesis is a ridiculous 37-step process, and since I value my friendships, I won't take you through all the steps. But below are a few things to help guide you along which will have some relevance when we eventually discuss DRUGS, BIOMARKERS, and the BRAIN: (Seriously, feel free to skip this for now and refer back to it later if you're starting to harbor resentment towards me).

1. The synthesis of cholesterol starts from a couple molecules of acetyl-CoA.
2. The "key enzyme" in the entire process is hydroxymethylglutaryl-CoA reductase, or HMG-CoA reductase, which you will know as the drug target of STATINS. Statins inhibit this step, thus decreasing cholesterol synthesis.
3. Eventually, the molecule gets so long that an intermediate called squalene forms a ring called lanosterol. From there, lanosterol has 2 different pathways.
4. Below the brain, lanosterol is converted primarily to LATHOSTEROL in what is known as the Kandutsch-Russell pathway.
5. In the brain, lanosterol is primarily converted to DESMOSTEROL in what is known as the Bloch pathway.
6. But, the end result regardless of the pathway is the production of cholesterol. There are just different precursors and different enzymes that catalyze the formation of the final product in each pathway.

Wow, that was energetically expensive to read through that, and so is the process of making cholesterol...it takes a TON of ATP to create this stuff, and that's partially why our bodies have a very sophisticated transport system that involves recycling and repurposing cholesterol as it serves its myriad of functions throughout the body. This provides a nice segway (yes I know it's technically *segue*, but I like the mental image of riding on a motorized scooter) into our next topic, the vitally important LIPOPROTEINS. But to make sure you're not drowning from the mini-deluge, just remind yourself of the essential core concepts from this section.

1. **A lack of cholesterol is incompatible with life**, and cholesterol serves a whole bunch of critical functions.
2. **Every nucleated cell in your body synthesizes its own cholesterol.** There is a tightly regulated sweet spot of cellular cholesterol...too little and you're not alive, too much and your cell explodes.

3

LIPOPROTEINS

Once again, as we embark on this discussion of lipoproteins, remember these axioms:

1. Blood is mostly water, and fat and water don't mix, so we need LIPOPROTEINS as the vehicles to transport LIPIDS, since they are WATER-SOLUBLE.
2. The purpose of these LIPOPROTEINS is NOT to give you heart disease. Lipoproteins are simply MAILMEN. Most mailmen are just regular citizens. Their job is to deliver the mail (triglycerides primarily) and then go home (to the liver) at the end of the day. However, if that mailman runs his truck into your arterial wall, which is how atherosclerosis starts, that mailman is a criminal and needs to be addressed.

What does it mean that lipoproteins are "low-density" or "high-density?"

Fat floats...we've all seen the guy at the pool party who weighs about 3 bills but displays remarkable buoyancy. In contrast, the gym bro who eats 400 grams of protein a day and has single-digit body fat percentage, tends to sink. Similarly, the density of a lipoprotein refers to whether or not it tends to sink in water. The higher the fat content in a lipoprotein, the greater the buoyancy. The higher the protein content of a lipoprotein, the higher the density.

The first type of lipoprotein we will consider is the **chylomicron.** Chylomicrons are intestinally produced and generally are only present after you eat. These could also be called "very very very low-density lipoproteins," but chylomicron sounds more sophisticated than VVVLDL. These guys have a ton of triglycerides on them and very little protein, and if you're using a centrifuge to separate these things in a chem lab, these tend to float to the top.

Very-low density lipoproteins (VLDL), **intermediate-density lipoproteins** (IDL), **and low-density lipoproteins** (LDL) are produced by the liver. VLDL still have a lot of triglycerides, but less than chylomicrons, and as you reach each subsequent density classification, the lipoprotein will have relatively fewer trigs but more cholesteryl ester and protein content. **High-density lipoprotein** (HDL) particles are the most prevalent, but also the smallest of the lipoprotein particles. Since HDL have the highest relative protein content, they sink. Not too bad, right?

Of note, each LDL particle carries about 2,200 molecules of cholesterol, while each HDL particle only carries about 45 under normal circumstances. That little pearl will become more meaningful later.

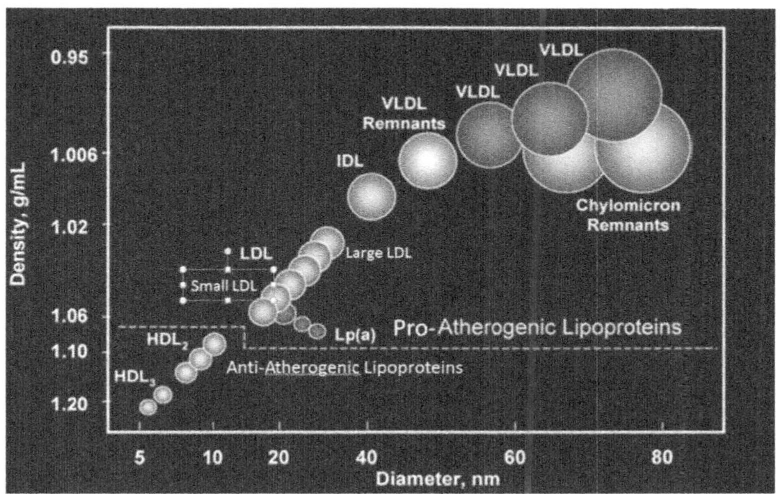

Figure 5: Lipoprotein Densities: Fat floats, so the big, fat triglyceride-rich chylomicrons have the lowest density, followed by chylomicron remnants and VLDL. The HDL particles, which have far fewer lipids and more relative protein content, "sink" compared to the other particles. Source: Feingold, K. R. (2024). Introduction to Lipids and Lipoproteins. In K.R. Feingold (Eds.) et. al., *Endotext*. MDText.com, Inc.

The ApoB Family

The ApoB family (B for Bad if they end up in your arterial wall) includes chylomicrons, chylomicron remnants, VLDL, IDL, LDL, and Lp(a) particles. Lp(a), which is the potential "felon" of the lipid neighborhood, serves a different function than these other mailmen, so it will receive its own special treatment in a later section. Aside from the fat and fluffy chylomicrons, there is potential for any of these particles to end up in your arterial wall, since any particle <70 nanometers in diameter is capable of getting into the wrong place. Size does matter, but the character of the particles matters a whole lot more (that's what I've been telling myself my whole life as a well-below average-sized person).

Chylomicrons differ from VLDL, IDL, and LDL particles in that they have an ApoB-48 molecule rather than an ApoB-100. The ApoB-48 tells us that it is intestinally derived, and the reason it's called ApoB-48 is because this truncated ApoB is 48% the molecular weight of ApoB-100. The mailmen with ApoB-48 on their name badges predominate in the postprandial period (after you eat), and don't really work the night shift (unless you're eating all night long, in which case you're certainly not controlling your insulin or life). In that case, there becomes a "traffic jam" of ApoB-48 and ApoB-100 molecules trying to get home to the liver; excess chylomicrons can compete for the clearance of other particles, which can become problematic.

So VLDL, IDL, and LDL particles, which are produced by the liver, are the mailmen that are consistently delivering the mail throughout the day, and they are characterized by an ApoB-100 molecule, which is 550 kilodaltons (kD) in molecular weight. This is significant for 3 reasons:

1. There is **one** ApoB-100 molecule on every one of these mailmen (VLDL, IDL, LDL).
2. That same ApoB-100 remains with that particle for its entire lifespan until it is cleared from the body.
3. We know the molecular weight of ApoB-100 is always 550 kD.

Given these axioms, employing ApoB as a lab metric gives us a more accurate picture of the PARTICLES in your neighborhood. Since PARTICLES determine the number of potential criminals in your lipid neighborhood, ApoB becomes a superior metric of lipid-mediated risk...more on that later in Chapter 7.

Conventionally, we are taught that VLDL particles dump off their triglycerides, then become IDLs, who then become LDLs. In general, most of the "potential criminals" in your neighborhood are LDLs, since they linger in your bloodstream for several days in contrast to chylomicrons, VLDL, and IDL. Much of this tendency to "loiter" by LDL particles is due to their lack of another apolipoprotein, ApoE (E for Easy access for liver clearance...more on that later). In contrast, chylomicrons and IDL are typically cleared within minutes, whereas VLDL particles generally hang around a few hours.

The primary determinant of ApoB-100 molecule production is the availability of triglycerides in the liver. Triglycerides primarily arrive at the liver via lipolysis (the liberation of fatty acids that have been stored in your "suitcases," the fat cells). There are 2 situations in which lipolysis could be happening: (1) in an insulin-sensitive condition, which is optimal, and (2) in an insulin-resistant (sub-optimal) physiologic state.

1. When you haven't eaten, which should be a condition of low insulin (the storage hormone), glucagon (the hormonal "opposite" of insulin) signals your fat cells to dump out their triglycerides...this is accessing your "savings account." Then your liver gets all this "mail," (triglycerides), and then the mailmen (the ApoB particles) deliver the mail, unload their cargo, and fuel your tissues before returning home (the liver) at the end of the day. Awesome!
2. BUT, when people are insulin resistant, the proper storage function of insulin is impaired, and your adipocyte suitcases are full anyway...no more room! So, LIPOLYSIS occurs even in a state WHEN IT SHOULDN'T. Insulin normally suppresses lipolysis, but your fat cells become "resistant" to its normal effects. The liver is flooded with even more triglycerides and shuttles out more ApoB mailmen to deliver all the mail. But wait...all the mailboxes are full (mixed my metaphors there, but hopefully you're tracking). So what are the mailmen going to do? Good question...there's a

lot of traffic out there, they can't deliver the mail since the mailboxes are full, and they JUST MIGHT RUN THEIR TRUCKS INTO YOUR ARTERIAL WALL. And that's one of the big reasons why we see a heightened risk of ASCVD in people with diabesity/insulin resistance/metabolic syndrome. Additionally, in conditions of elevated blood sugars, the mailmen can get caught in a "sugar storm" and become GLYCATED. It's tough to drive safely in a storm, and an ApoB particle that becomes glycated (basically bound up by sugar), is much more likely to crash your arterial wall.

a. If the mailboxes are full and the mailmen aren't going home, you end up having a bunch of TRIGLYCERIDE-RICH REMNANTS. As stated previously, normally a VLDL particle delivers the mail, and then after he delivers some mail becomes an IDL. And then the IDL goes home to the liver or delivers a little more mail and becomes an LDL. (Sometimes LDL are secreted directly from the liver as well without first being a VLDL/IDL). BUT, if the VLDL or IDL doesn't go home, they are called **remnants** and are about 4 times as likely to cause heart disease than your run-of-the mill LDL particle.
b. You may have heard of the "small dense LDL particle", or sd-LDL. Now, as I said, any of these particles are small enough to get into the subendothelial space of your arterial intima where they don't belong (LDL particles are 18-23 nanometers in diameter and any particle <70 nm can infiltrate the vessel). And particle for particle, the sdLDL seems more likely to be retained in the artery. But in this case, I would say that size really doesn't matter...the atherogenicity of the small LDL

particle is more due to its "character." These sdLDL are more enriched in an amino acid called lysine, which has a POSITIVE charge. And there are components of the inner artery lining called heparan sulfate proteoglycans (HSPGs), which have a NEGATIVE charge. Basically, it's like a magnet; the sdLDL sticks in the artery, and then the process of plaque formation ensues. Additionally, sdLDL are more likely to have something called ApoC3, which is basically "the great inhibitor" of particle clearance. And if the particles loiter, they are more likely to cause mischief, as we've discussed at length.

c. And where do we typically see a bunch of sdLDL and ApoC3? You guessed it...insulin resistance.
d. BONUS ROUND: The very SMALLEST of the LDL particles is called electronegative L5 LDL...it's actually between the size of an HDL and an LDL. Given what I just said about the "magnetic" effect of sdLDL tending to "stick" in the artery, this electronegativity may seem counterintuitive. But, we all know that, outside of some rare sociopaths, crimes tend to be COMMMITTED IN GROUPS, and L5 LDL are very prone to AGGREGATION. And so they collectively wreak havoc on your endothelial cells. And what situations do we most commonly see these nefarious LDL gangs with super bad Little-man Syndrome? Yep, diabetes, smoking, and chronic inflammatory conditions.

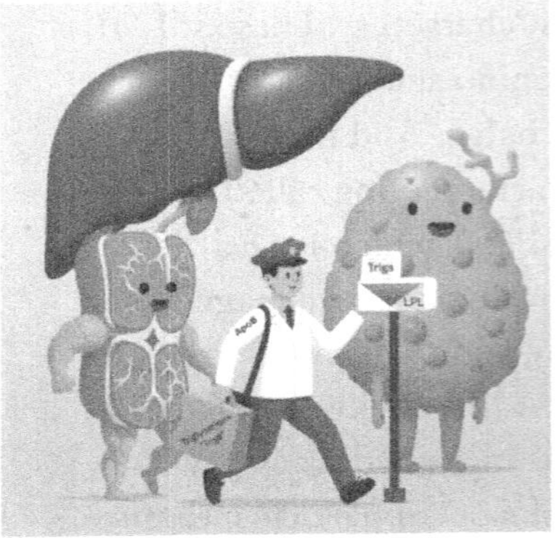

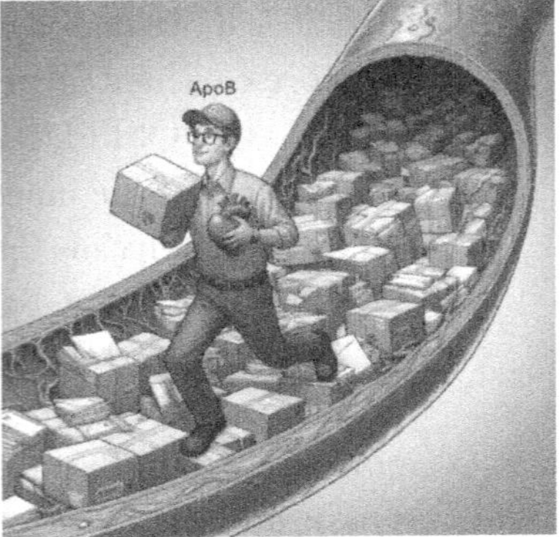

Figure 6: The "Good Mailman" and the "Mailman Gone Rogue." On the left we see the ApoB mailman delivering the triglyceride mail into the LPL mailbox of the fat and muscle cells before he returns "home" to the liver at the end of his shift. On the right, we see the criminalized ApoB mailman who has been delivering his cholesterol and triglyceride cargo into an arterial wall, and the "plaque-ages" are already building up!

So to recap:

- **ApoB-48 chylomicron mailmen from the intestine predominate after you've eaten and typically aren't around when you're fasting...**but if they're around in excess they can cause **a traffic jam** and compete for clearance with the ApoB-100 particles.
- **If ApoB particles AREN'T delivering the mail** (primarily triglycerides) to muscle cells or fat cells due to either a traffic jam, full mailboxes, or both, **then they are much more likely to crash into your arterial wall where they don't belong.**
- **It's more about the CHARACTER of the particle than the SIZE when it comes to potentially getting into the arterial wall.** Any of the ApoB particles can get in, but remnants and sdLDL have some unique properties that make them more likely to loiter and never make it home to the liver.

Major Players in Clearance

Ok, so we've discussed the importance of CLEARANCE of these potential criminals, which really are just mailmen. But we need to have an understanding of HOW this process occurs, and the **major means by which these ApoB-100 particles are cleared is the LOW-DENSITY LIPOPROTEIN RECEPTOR (LDLr) in the liver.** ApoB-48 is cleared by a different receptor called the LDL receptor-related protein 1 (LRP1), and since, in general, the majority of the ApoB that we see in circulation are of the ApoB-100 variety, we will focus on LDLr.

I like to visualize the LDLr as one of those coin-operated "claw grabbers" that you see at the arcade when you try to win your kids a stuffed animal. The LDLr is the claw, and it recognizes the ApoB on the stuffed animal, grabs it, and pulls it in. YES! And you win your kid the stuffed animal, everyone is happy, and the next parents gets in line to win their kid a stuffed animal. Under normal circumstances, this is what occurs; the LDLr can recirculate hundreds of times and pull in the LDL particles, which then get degraded in the lysosome (which is essentially the cellular garbage disposal). Although the lipoprotein is degraded, the cholesterol can be recycled for other cellular functions and the claw grabber stays in working order.

UNLESS, a protein called **proprotein convertase subtilisin kexin type 9** (PCSK9) comes around (you know you've earned your lipid stripes when you can flawlessly enunciate PCSK9's full name without sounding like you're puking). **PCSK9 puts the LDLR CLAW GRABBER OUT OF COMMISSION**.

Instead of recirculating to the cell surface, the LDLr bound by PCSK9 is degraded in the lysosome along with the LDL particle. Oh no! And people are still getting in line, but the claw grabber is out of order. Kids are crying, stuffed animals aren't being won,

LDL particles aren't being cleared, and PEOPLE ARE GETTING HEART DISEASE.

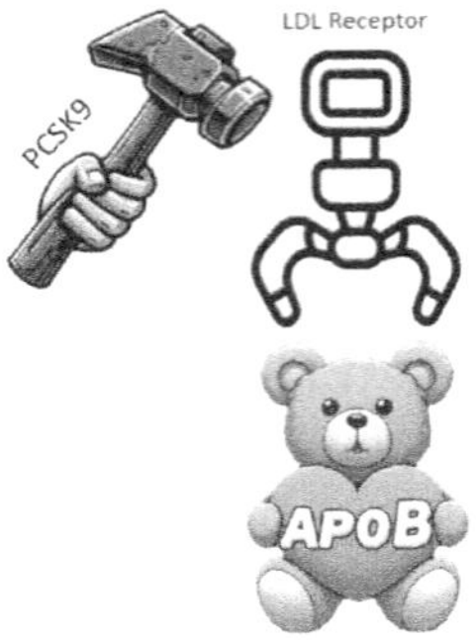

Figure 7: Major players in lipoprotein clearance.
The LDLr "claw grabber" wins the ApoB Bear UNLESS PCSK9 puts the LDLr claw grabber "out of order."

Familial Hypercholesterolemia (FH)

Now that you know the major players in clearance, a brief discussion of FAMILIAL HYPERCHOLESTEROLEMIA, or FH, will make a lot more sense, since the gene mutations involved in FH are ***LDLR, APOB,*** or ***PCSK9.***

FH can come in 2 different flavors: HOMOZYGOUS FH and HETEROZYGOUS FH. FH is what's called an autosomal dominant condition...if you have one copy of a certain gene, then you will have high cholesterol levels (an LDL-c >190) no matter what you do. And if you have 2 copies of that gene, your cholesterol levels will be stratospheric, usually an LDL-c >500.

Homozygous FH is a terrible disease that reiterates the concept that sometimes you just need to "pick the right parents." These poor kids end up having their first heart attacks by age 10 and are in and out of the coronary cath lab throughout most of their lives. And it isn't because they have an impaired Home Security

System; they certainly are not insulin resistant, hypertensive, inflamed, or smoking. But their Lipid Neighborhood is so dangerous that they get "broken into" very early in life.

Evinacumab to the Rescue!
HoFH is a HORRIBLE DISEASE, and since most lipid-lowering pharmaceuticals act by increasing the LDL receptor claw-grabbers, they really don't work particularly well in HoFH (since these people basically have zero claw grabbers to begin with). However, Evinacumab, which is an ANGPTL3 inhibitor (more on that in the Deep Dive on the ANGPTL family) works to clear ApoB particles by non-LDL receptor pathways, lowering LDL-c by around 50% in those with HoFH.

People with Heterozygous FH (HeFH) often get early and advanced heart disease as well, but there are some who seem to escape this fate, which is interesting. In general, these folks with HeFH who avoid coronary disease have perfect Home Security Systems, and I believe they ought to be studied in detail to see if they possess other protective features. We often learn more from the exceptions than the rule in biology. And not everyone with an LDL-c >190 has one of the known autosomal dominant alleles...much more to learn.

But, if you have genetically confirmed FH, now that we know that LDLr, ApoB, and PCSK9 are critical factors in CLEARANCE, the following should make sense:

- ***LDLR* mutation** = Less LDLr Claw Grabbers. Less LDLr Claw Grabbers = More LDL particles. More LDL particles = More potential for the LDL particles to cause mischief since they're not being cleared.
- ***APOB* mutation** = The stuffed animals (particles) that would normally be picked up by the LDLr claw grabbers keep slipping out, since the ApoB is not "recognized" by the LDLr. The line gets longer, nobody is winning the

stuffed animals, and we, once again, have MORE LDL PARTICLES and less clearance.

- ***PCSK9* mutation** = This is actually a GAIN-OF-FUNCTION mutation in which there is TOO MUCH PCSK9 around. And we know that PCSK9 "puts your LDLr claw grabbers out of order." The end result is the same...less LDLr claw grabbers means more LDL particles and more potential for heart disease.

GOLIATH has a nice RING to it

Although PCSK9 is the most well-known regulator of LDL receptor activity, there are some other minority regulators that influence clearance of lipoproteins. Although certainly not worthy of anyone's worship, there is a protein called IDOL (Inducible Degrader of Low-Density Lipoprotein Receptor) that is influenced by the sterol sensor LXR. Basically, when LXR senses too many sterols inside the cell, specifically oxysterols, it activates IDOL to limit the amount of LDL receptors that recycle to the cell surface. But really the entire reason I'm writing this section is an excuse to talk about my favorite regulator of LDL receptor activity, an E3 ubiquitin ligase called GOLIATH. So GOLIATH is ironically quite small and probably not very influential, but it does seem to play a similar role to IDOL in regulating LDL receptor expression. But the best part about GOLIATH is that in order for it to work, it depends on a protein domain called a RING. You may be thinking, "Oh, I bet it has a circular shape...that makes sense." But you'd be SO WRONG...the truth is far more hilarious...RING is an acronym for Really Interesting New Gene...you can't make this stuff up! And this is my motivation for trying to learn these things, in hopes that I can discover a new protein and then name it something ridiculous so that I can laugh about it with my three or four similarly deranged friends.

So to recap what we learn from FH:

- **People with Homozygous FH** live in such a rough Lipid Neighborhood that, no matter their Home Security System, they **will get broken into early and often.** This reinforces the axiom that you CANNOT have atherosclerosis without an ApoB lipoprotein infiltrating your arterial wall.

- The main players in LDL clearance are the **LDLr and PCSK9**. The LDLr is like the claw grabber at the arcade, and it keeps working beautifully unless PCSK9 binds to it and puts it "out of order." The less particle clearance, the more particles that may wind up in your arterial wall.

4

HDL: THE "GOOD" CHOLESTEROL

"A static plasma measurement of HDL cholesterol gives you NO IDEA of its functionality."
-A bunch of people who know some stuff about lipids

At this point we've established that the label of "good cholesterol" or "bad cholesterol" is preposterous. It's the same cholesterol molecule; it's just a matter of where it's at and where it's going. But I'll just briefly give you a few main concepts about high-density lipoproteins (For those who want a deeper dive on HDL, you will have that opportunity in the next section).

1. The primary apolipoprotein on HDL particles is ApoA-1, and there are between 1 and 5 of these ApoA-1 particles on each HDL particle.
2. Although low HDL-c is associated with increased risk of heart disease (usually due to insulin resistance, which will mechanistically be further explained in the subsequent chapter), there are many people with normal or high HDL-c who also have heart disease. In fact, the trend for people with very high HDL-c levels seems to

be in the WRONG direction in regards to mortality (but not always). And trying to engineer drugs to raise HDL have failed EVERY SINGLE TIME in regards to reducing cardiovascular events. And remember what alcohol does to HDL? Yep, raises it...and I'd love to hear the argument that the HDL-raising effect of alcohol is somehow beneficial.

3. HDL is capable of performing a bunch of awesome functions throughout the body. HDL can take a cholesterol-laden ApoB perpetrator in the arterial wall and transport it back to the liver in a process called cholesterol efflux capacity (CEC). If you're having a particularly bad day and end up with sepsis, HDL can serve as a sink for toxins such as lipopolysaccharides (LPS) and these poisons can eventually be excreted in the bile in a process called Reverse LPS Transport. And HDL can even enhance glucose uptake in skeletal muscle. These are all good things, but calling it "good cholesterol" is still inaccurate. **A random blood measurement cannot tell you whether or not the HDL is doing anything good or bad.**
4. HDL is super complicated and harbors hundreds of proteins that may contribute to its functionality or dysfunctionality. People with autoimmune diseases sometimes have dysfunctional HDL particles, and glycated HDL (if caught in a sugar storm) seems to have less antioxidant and "damage control" proteins. But once again, who knows? It's inaccurate and dangerous to think you're invincible just because your HDL-c on your labwork is high and any ratio involving HDL "looks good."

If we continue our Home Security System and Lipid Neighborhood metaphor, the HDL particles can be considered "policemen" who are capable of arriving at the crime scene where an ApoB mailman has crashed his truck into your artery. **The HDL can help clean up the mess, take the criminal into custody, and return him to the jail cells of the liver**. Sometimes they can keep the well-meaning inflammatory citizens from making the crime scene worse. And the HDL cops can contribute to a bunch of other beneficial community activities as well. But sometimes they become fat with triglycerides and get removed from the police force, and maybe they get caught in sugar storm traffic, and sometimes they may "look good" on the surface but end up being corrupt. We just don't know by looking at the community census or police reports, which would be your cholesterol panel. The snapshot of HDL levels in your blood doesn't tell us much about what's happening in the actual physiologic movie, ergo:

> **ApoE for EMERGENCY**
>
> ApoE, best known for its role in clearance of triglyceride-rich lipoproteins as well as lipid transport in the brain, can also be produced by macrophages. When macrophages produce ApoE, particularly at the "scene of a crime" in the arterial wall, it essentially functions as an "Emergency Alarm" so that HDL particles can come in and hopefully evict the sterol-laden miscreant from the arterial intima.

"A static plasma measurement of HDL cholesterol gives you NO IDEA of its functionality."

5

CHOLESTEROL PATHWAYS

AND REVERSE CHOLESTEROL TRANSPORT-MASTERS CLASS EDITION

"If you tell me I can't do something, I can't wait to prove you wrong."
-Brooks Koepka (also my ploy to possibly get you to read this chapter, at least eventually)

Remember those "Choose Your Own Adventure" books? You would read a chapter and then be faced with a dilemma...choose the "right" path and you would earn the chance to see the plot unfold. Choose the "wrong" path and the next chapter would abruptly end in you being dismembered or being eaten by a hippo. I read about 54 of these books when I was in second grade as part of a contest to earn a free personal pan pizza at Pizza Hut; these are the things we used to do prior to video games. But there was this one kid named Danny who would find the shortest route to "finishing" each one of these books by discovering the path that ended in a premature ending without exploring all the other possible options. Then he would say he "completed another book" and ended up earning his pizza way before the rest of us. Truly Breakfast of Champion-type behavior.

But at this point, I'm giving you the option to "Pull a Danny." In this section we will discuss what are referred to as the ENDOGENOUS and EXOGENOUS pathways of cholesterol transport as well as REVERSE CHOLESTEROL TRANSPORT. If you're a medical student you probably ought to stick around. And if you want to understand why dietary cholesterol, in general, has very little impact on your blood cholesterol and what really happens in your body when you eat an egg, you can skip to the EXOGENOUS pathway section. And if you want a deep dive into HDL biology and REVERSE CHOLESTEROL TRANSPORT, by all means skip to that section. But feel free to forge ahead...even if you skip this chapter, I'd still let you claim that you read the book.

The Endogenous Pathway

Although this pathway represents a small fraction of TOTAL body cholesterol synthesis since every cell and tissue in your body creates its own, the cholesterol from this pathway is the MAJORITY of what we would see on your cholesterol panel, usually around 85% or so.

And this is the classic "ApoB-100" pathway which states that VLDL becomes an IDL which becomes an LDL. We've discussed this, and I'll review the steps briefly below:

1. You've got some triglycerides (mail) in the liver.
2. Your liver creates an apoprotein (ApoB) which becomes an apolipoprotein when it acquires lipids. ApoB-100 (the mailman) needs to deliver the mail (triglycerides and a few phospholipids), and this mailman carrying the mail is a VLDL particle.
3. Along the way, an HDL graciously provides guidance for the ApoB-100 VLDL on where to deliver the mail (ApoC2) and a GPS/access card to make sure he can

easily get home at the end of the day (ApoE, E for EASY, since particles with ApoE are easily recognized by the LDLr for clearance).

4. The mailman (VLDL ApoB-100) delivers the mail (primarily triglycerides) to muscle cells (including heart muscle cells), or fat cells, and the triglycerides get into these cells via LPL (lipoprotein lipase). ApoC2 helps facilitate LPL activity.
5. Once he (the VLDL) delivers the mail, he now has fewer triglycerides, so the mailman delivering a little less mail is now called an IDL.
6. About half of the IDLs go home to the liver and are cleared, but then some of them lose a few more triglycerides as well as that ApoE access card and become LDL particles. Since LDL particles no longer have ApoE, they have a longer half-life of about 2 days, meaning they stick around in your circulation for much longer.
7. Ideally, the LDL particles eventually go home to the liver and are cleared via the LDL receptor. Although the LDL lacks ApoE for Easy clearance, it still has ApoB, so this is how it eventually obtains hepatic access via the LDLr.

And then, when that cholesterol is in the liver, it has a few options:

1. The cholesterol can be used to create a bile acid or it can be sent out into the bile...remember, you can't make bile acids without a cholesterol precursor!
2. The cholesterol can be used to make a lipoprotein and "do it all over again."
3. The cholesterol can be stored, or ESTERIFIED, and saved for later.

It's all tightly regulated, primarily by a "sensor" called the sterol regulatory element binding protein (SREBP2) since a lack of cholesterol is incompatible with life, and too much cholesterol is toxic. If cholesterol is relatively "low" inside the cell and "needs more" then it can primarily take care of this problem by a couple of ways:

1. Increase LDL receptors to pull more cholesterol into the cell (more claw grabbers).
2. Increase production of cholesterol (via HMG-CoA reductase).

Once the liver is satisfied with its cholesterol collection, it decreases its own production and decreases the amount of LDL receptors. As long as this process is in happy equilibrium, everyone's happy, no one's cells are exploding, no one's liver is drenched in fatty sterol gravy, and no one's getting heart disease.

The Exogenous Pathway

Whenever I go to a cardiology conference, there will inevitably be someone who, at breakfast, feels guilty about eating scrambled eggs and makes some comment about the irony of it all. So even though, in general, this pathway represents a VERY SMALL fraction of your plasma cholesterol (around 15%), the intent of this section is to make you feel confident that, (unless you're what we call a "hyper-absorber" of dietary cholesterol), you can truly enjoy one of the most delicious and healthy foods on the planet without it meaningfully affecting your cholesterol bloodwork.

So here's what happens when you eat an egg, since we know the yolk has a TON of cholesterol, which we've all been taught to approach with trepidation:

1. The cholesterol in the egg is in its ESTERIFIED form, and your body has to DE-ESTERIFY it in order for it to even make it into your gut cell, which is called the enterocyte. It's kind of a lot of work, so most of the time that enzyme (called carboxyl ester lipase) just doesn't even bother.
   a. So you just poop it out.
2. But, let's say that you expend the effort to de-esterify the cholesterol in the egg yolk. Bile and other pancreatic enzymes come in to mulch up everything else that might be useful to have around and it creates something called a MICELLE. A micelle kind of looks like one of those holiday cheese balls and has cholesterol, fatty acids, some vitamins and other stuff in it which can now be available for uptake into the intestinal cell.
3. So there is a "cholesterol party" in the gut (kudos to Dr. Tom Dayspring here, the Lipid Legend from whom I first heard this analogy), and there is a "ticket taker" to the cholesterol party. The ticket taker's name is **Niemann-Pick C1-Like 1, or NPC1L1** from here on out. If you flash your sterol I.D., NPC1L1 lets you in and everyone is having a great time in the enterocyte.
4. But we know that intracellular, or "intra-party" cholesterol is tightly regulated, and there are a couple of guys watching the cameras in the party. These are the sterol-regulatory element binding proteins (SREBPs) and the liver X receptors (the nomenclature is confusing, but don't worry, there's a bunch of LXRs everywhere, not just the liver). They are watching closely to make sure the party isn't getting too crazy.
5. The moment there are a few too many cholesterol partygoers, the "bouncer" is activated, whose name is **ABCG5/G8** (I think **"A Buff Cop"** for **ABC**, which is who you want on patrol). He kicks out the excess sterols back into your gut lumen, where you poop them out.

6. Other sterols might find companionship at the party and can become part of an HDL particle, and others might be "mailmen" who need to go to work who become part of a chylomicron and leave the party through the thoracic duct as part of an ApoB-48 particle.

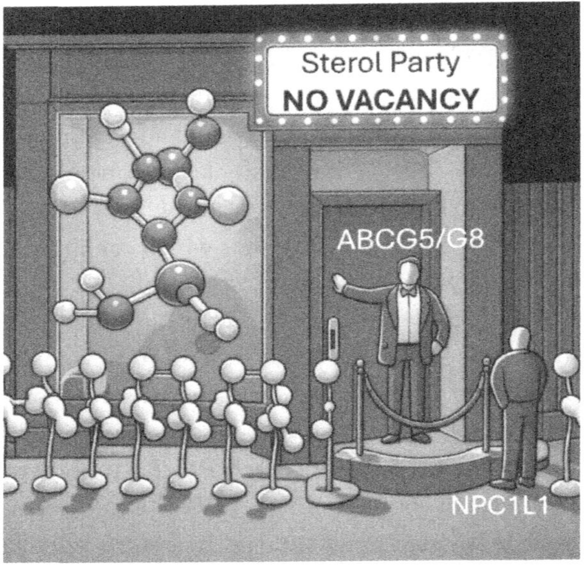

Figure 8: Cholesterol Regulation in the Intestine. NPC1L1 is the "ticket taker" to the sterol party, and ABCG5/G8 is the "bouncer" if the party gets a little too crazy, evicting rowdy sterols into the nearest toilet bowl.

So to recap the main points here:

- **NPC1L1** is the "ticket taker" to the cholesterol party in the gut cell.
- **ABCG5/G8** is the "bouncer" if there are too many cholesterol partygoers.

- The whole process is tightly regulated, so unless your ticket taker is very undiscerning and/or your bouncers are off duty, whatever dietary cholesterol you ingest won't usually affect your blood levels hardly at all.

This is important to know because we have a cholesterol drug, called *Ezetimibe*, which inhibits NPC1L1. Its mechanism of action is to make your ticket-taker more discriminate. Take Ezetimibe, and your ticket-taker doesn't let as many sterols into the party. Makes sense, right?

There are always exceptions in lipidology, but in general, dietary cholesterol has very little impact on your blood cholesterol. So logically, Ezetimibe isn't very potent compared to other methods of lowering cholesterol unless the individual tends to be a hyper-absorber of these sterols. Cool stuff!

Reverse Cholesterol Transport, HDL, and CETP

Let's start with the "textbook" definitions of Reverse Cholesterol Transport, and then we will embark on an odyssey of sorts that will be well worth the crusade...this part will get a little granular, but there will be so many light bulbs going off in your head it may result in a full-blown epiphany if you see it through.

Classically, it is taught that Reverse Cholesterol Transport can be DIRECT or INDIRECT. Direct reverse cholesterol transport is when an HDL particle drops off its cholesterol cargo at the liver (often via a receptor called Scavenger Receptor B1, or SR-B1). Indirect reverse cholesterol transport is when the HDL particle gives its cholesterol to an LDL particle and then it gets delivered to the liver via the LDL receptor. (There is also a pathway called TICE, or trans-intestinal cholesterol efflux, that eliminates cholesterol via direct gut delivery, but it's poorly understood at this time so we'll skip it in this edition).

This exchange process is regulated in large part by a protein called cholesteryl ester transfer protein, or **CETP.** Here's how it works:

1. The HDL particle donates its cholesterol to the LDL particle via CETP, which basically creates a tunnel between the particles. In exchange, the HDL takes the triglycerides from the LDL. It's sort of like if you've ever gone to the bank drive-through and used the cool pneumatic tube thing to complete your transaction.
2. In conditions of triglyceride excess (ahem, insulin resistance), the HDL particle keeps accepting all the trigs and giving away its cholesterol.
3. The HDL particle is NOT supposed to be all "fat and fluffy" with triglycerides, so a couple of different enzymes called lipases come in and try to trim the fat, so to speak.
4. But after trimming the fat off the HDL, it becomes apparent that there's a pathetic, gaunt, emaciated HDL particle that's no good for anything. So your kidney actually gets involved and takes it out of circulation.
5. **This is why INSULIN RESISTANCE** (or metabolic syndrome or diabetes) **is associated with LOW HDL CHOLESTEROL.** Too many triglycerides around, a ton of CETP activity, and a whole bunch of bloated HDL particles that end up dying in the attempted fat removal procedure.
6. As stated previously, the static blood level of HDL-c gives you NO IDEA of its functionality. But, as HDL gurus like Dan Rader have said, if you're going to use HDL-c for anything from your bloodwork **it's kind of like the HbA1c of triglyceride levels.** If your triglyceride levels are chronically high (even if your fasting levels are normal), your HDL-c will become lower over time. (There are exceptions to this as well, as

insulin resistant populations of African ancestry will often have normal HDL and triglyceride levels).

HDL biology is PHENOMENALLY COMPLICATED, and the basics have been delineated previously. But for you who are interested in a slightly deeper dive, I'm going to shift my metaphor from mailmen and home security to sports, specifically American football (I love all sports...I played college baseball and ran intercollegiate track, but I was neither mean enough, tough enough, nor large enough to ever set foot on the gridiron):

1. **HDL is like a quarterback**. In contrast to the ApoB family of lipoproteins, the main structural apolipoprotein on HDL is ApoA-1, and there are between 1 and 5 ApoA-1s on each HDL. And in contrast to the ApoB family, HDL particles start off smaller in size. And when HDL is "young" he's just a scrawny, frisbee-shaped particle who really needs to mature in order to develop into a useful team leader.
2. In order for the young HDL to mature, he needs to be coachable, and he needs others to impart teaching and wisdom. **The intrinsic coachability in our young quarterback is lecithin cholesterol acyltransferase, or LCAT**, which allows him to esterify cholesterol; without it, he can never develop (that's why those with LCAT deficiency have almost non-existent HDL levels). Then the young HDL acquires cholesterol via ABCA1 and, as he further develops, ABCG1. With this "experience" he can then do all the tasks required of a Cholesterol Quarterback.
3. Now, the HDL Quarterback can help his teammates out, donating other lipoproteins such as ApoC2 and ApoE to his teammates (ApoB particles), which will help them perform their jobs more effectively. And he

himself is capable of "quarterback sneaking" his way into the Liver End Zone, which is analogous to DIRECT REVERSE CHOLESTEROL TRANSPORT.

a. However, quarterback sneaks are generally only good for 1 yard, so the liver cannot satisfy its intracellular cholesterol demand merely by this mechanism since each HDL particle only has about 45 molecules of cholesterol**. BUT, the HDL quarterback can complete long passes via CETP to his LDL wide receivers,** and they can score 70 yard touchdowns (because each LDL particle has around 2200 molecules of cholesterol each) **in the INDIRECT REVERSE CHOLESTEROL TRANSPORT** process. Of course, the LDL wide-receivers can always "fumble" into your arterial wall, but ideally that won't happen.

4. Still though, just by "looking" at your HDL cholesterol, we can't tell if he's a good quarterback. Most "short" quarterbacks are going to struggle, and usually low HDL-c is indicative of some metabolic issues (but not always). If the HDL possesses certain proteins such as ApoC3 or serum amyloid A, he's going to be a dysfunctional quarterback, even if he seems "prototypical on paper." And there are a variety of genetic mutations that result in high but dysfunctional HDL-c levels and accelerated heart disease.

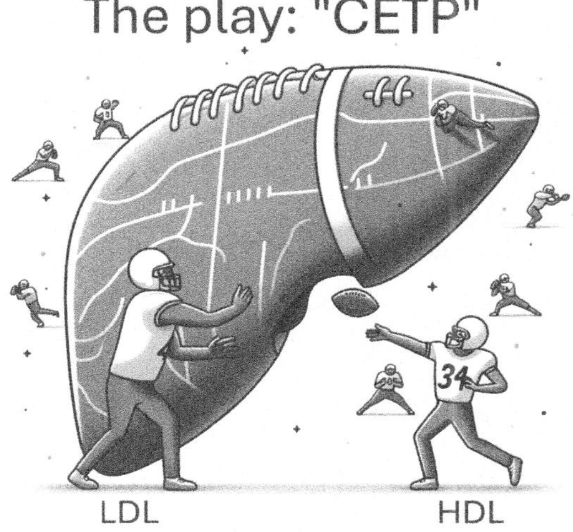

Figure 9: CETP-mediated Reverse Cholesterol Transport. The HDL quarterback can either score short touchdowns in the Liver End Zone himself (Direct Reverse Cholesterol Transport) or, via CETP, pass the cholesterol football to LDL wide receivers for long scoring plays (Indirect Reverse Cholesterol Transport).

So to recap:

- **HDL is like a quarterback** who can either "score" in the liver end zone by a quarterback sneak (DIRECT) or via CETP "pass the ball" to an ApoB wide receiver (typically LDL) for the touchdown (INDIRECT REVERSE CHOLESTEROL TRANSPORT) as depicted above.
- Most low HDL levels are due to insulin resistance, but **high HDL levels give you no idea of your HDL Quarterback's functionality;** there are many people with high HDL-c with advanced vascular disease.

And as a prize for reading this "optional" chapter, you get a cool chart that will help you review selected apolipoproteins and their functions on the next page! (Recall that apoproteins become apolipoproteins when they acquire lipids, which should make sense).

Table 1: Selected Peripheral Apolipoproteins

Apolipoprotein	**Lipoprotein Association**	**Function(s)**	**English, Please! Purpose in the Lipid Neighborhood**
ApoA1	HDL, Prechylomicron	LCAT activator Mediates ABCA1/ABCG1 efflux Primary lipoprotein on HDL	The badge of the HDL policemen, gives the HDL its identity.
ApoA5	VLDL	Activates LPL when insulin levels are low	Helps the mailmen deliver the mail.
ApoB-48	Chylomicron	Postprandial lipid transport Ligand for LRP1 Produced by the intestine	Mailmen that only work the "after you eat" shift
ApoB-100	VLDL, IDL, LDL, Lp(a)	Lipid transport Ligand for LDLr Produced by the liver	Mailmen that work around the clock
ApoC1	HDL, VLDL	LCAT activator LPL inhibitor CETP inhibitor Smallest of the lipoproteins	He's little and mysterious! Don't worry about it for now.
ApoC2	HDL, chylomicrons, VLDL	LPL activator	Helps the mailmen deliver the mail.
ApoC3	HDL, chylomicrons, VLDL, LDL	LPL inhibitor Retards remnant clearance	"The great inhibitor" Prevents the mailmen from "going home"
ApoE	HDL, chylomicrons, VLDL, IDL	Triglyceride hydrolysis Regulates remnant clearance	Access code for the mailmen to get home to the liver
Apo(a)	Lp(a)	Unknown Lp(a) an independent risk factor for ASCVD	"The Felon among Criminals in the Lipid Neighborhood"

6

LP(A): THE "FELON" OF THE LIPID NEIGHBORHOOD

"The more you know, the more you realize you don't know."
-Aristotle, probably in reference to lipids

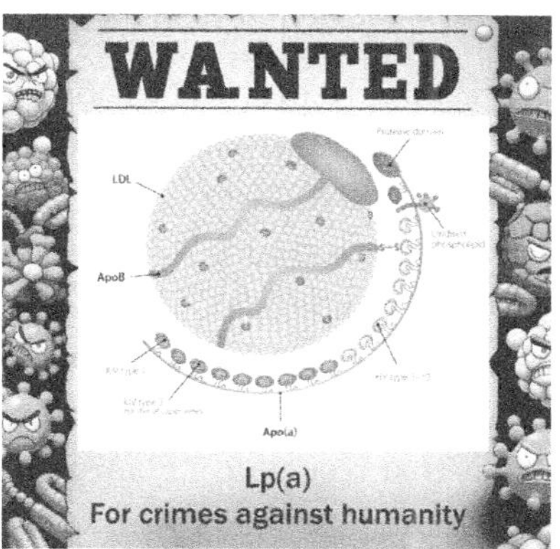

Figure 10: Lp(a): The "Felon" of the Lipid Neighborhood. Source: Svilaas, T., Klemsdal, T. O., Bogsrud, M. P., Græsdal, A., Vesterbekkmo, E. K., Asprusten, E. A., Langslet, G., & Retterstøl, K. (2022). High levels of lipoprotein(a): Assessment and treatment. *Tidsskrift for den Norske laegeforening: Tidsskrift for praktisk medicin, ny raekke*, *142*(1), 10.4045/tidsskr.21.0800. https://doi.org/10.4045/tidsskr.21.0800

So you'll remember back when we began this journey that I mentioned the "felon" of the Lipid Neighborhood as something called "Lp(a)." And I've specifically waited until now to discuss this unique lipoprotein, because it really isn't a mailman like the other ApoB-containing lipoproteins. But it certainly can "go rogue" and wreak havoc in your arterial wall...**for every 50 extra Lp(a) particles in your neighborhood, it carries a 28% increased risk of a break-in**...compare that with a 4% increased risk for every 50 extra run-of-the mill LDL. So it certainly can be a bad guy, and just like some of the worst criminals, it's rather mysterious; we've known about Lp(a) since 1963 and STILL DON'T KNOW HOW IT'S CLEARED FROM THE BODY...or really why it exists at all. But in the following question-and-answer format, I'll give you the important things to know about this independent risk factor for cardiovascular disease.

1. **What is Lp(a)?**
    a. Lp(a) is NOT an LDL particle, although it is often said to be "LDL-like" since it has one ApoB-100. However, this ApoB-100 is "married" to an apo(a) in the liver and then goes out into the body as an unhappy couple. This apo(a), which is COMPLETELY different than the ApoA-1 on HDL particles, has a bunch of protein domains called Kringles on it that resemble a Danish pastry; it is similar in structure to something else called *plasminogen*. The amount of Lp(a) that you produce is dictated by the *LPA* gene on Chromosome 6, right next to the gene that codes for plasminogen. This gene is fully expressed by age 2.
2. **What is its purpose?**
    a. Great question. It seems to be involved in tissue healing. People with keloids, which are exaggeratedly

raised scars, seem to have higher Lp(a) levels. Growth hormone, which is known to accelerate tissue remodeling, also increases Lp(a) levels. It is commonly theorized to have been "extra insurance" for when hemorrhage was a more common way to die, but since we aren't regularly being mauled by tigers anymore, Lp(a) now finds other ways to ruin our lives. Maybe you should ask a hedgehog this question...it's the only non-primate that has Lp(a).

3. **So it sounds like a genetic issue...how common is it?**
   a. 1 in 5 people have elevated Lp(a) levels, making it VERY COMMON, and certain ethnicities have higher average levels than others. People of African ancestry have an average of 75 nmol/L, while those of Caucasian descent have a mean of 19 nmol/L.
4. **So what constitutes an "elevated" Lp(a) level?**
   a. If measured in mg/dL, *50 mg/dL* is considered high, and if measured in nmol/L, *125 nmol/L* is considered elevated. However, there appears to be increased risk of cardiovascular events starting at 30 mg/dL. The Bogalusa and Young Finns heart studies measured Lp(a) in children and then followed them through adolescence into early adulthood. And those with levels over 30 mg/dL had about a twofold increased risk of premature cardiovascular disease.
5. **This is confusing...why are we using different measurements?**
   a. Great question...we need to eventually all use *nmol/L*, which is a measure of PARTICLES, since, just like the other ApoB members, the NUMBER OF PARTICLES DETERMINES RISK. This is particularly important for Lp(a), since the molecular weight can vary from 180 to 800 kD...this is a pretty

big variance in contrast to every other ApoB particle, which are all 550 kD. And it's the "skinny guys" (the low molecular weight Lp(a) particles) that seem to the sneakiest and most incorrigible felons.

6. **What is its association with cardiovascular events?**
   a. People with the highest Lp(a) levels have a 2-3 fold risk of heart attacks and aortic stenosis along with increased risk of heart failure, peripheral artery disease, strokes in younger people, and possibly even kidney disease. Other than that, it's pretty harmless.
   b. A recent study even showed a link between elevated Lp(a) in the first trimester of pregnancy and preeclampsia along with increased risk of other complications such as intrauterine growth restriction. It takes a truly incorrigible delinquent to prey on mothers and their unborn children, but Lp(a) apparently is that type of criminal.
7. **So why is it so bad?**
   a. Well, Lp(a) is said to be PROTHROMBOTIC, PROINFLAMMATORY, and PROATHEROSCLEROTIC.
      i. PROTHROMBOTIC-Recall that Lp(a) resembles plasminogen. Plasminogen functions as an important "clot buster" in your body. If you bleed, you make a clot, and then the clot dissolves. But if the clots are forming in your arteries, that's how things like heart attacks and strokes occur. It was popular at one point to say that Lp(a) directly "inhibits plasminogen." This isn't exactly true, but proteins on Lp(a) such as histidine-rich glycoprotein are messing with your normal clot dissolution system somehow.
      ii. PROINFLAMMATORY-Lp(a) seems to bring with it many inflammatory cells once it "breaks

in" to your arterial wall, and the *LPA* gene itself can be stimulated by that interleukin IL-6 (remember him)? Additionally, Lp(a) carries inherently inflammatory particles such as alpha-1 acid glycoprotein, which just by the name sounds pretty sinister.

iii. PROATHEROSCLEROTIC-on that Kringle domain, specifically the 10th segment of Kringle 4 (KIV-10), there are OXIDIZED PHOSPHOLIPIDS. The entire process is complicated, but the end result of these oxidized phospholipids, which have very high affinity for the aortic valve, is the upregulation of an osteoblastic cascade. What does that mean for normal people? BONE in the AORTA. That should strike you as a bad thing. And if any "bone-like" substance is in your arteries, that's not a great thing for optimal blood flow. The table below summarizes the significance of the dastardly Danishes on Lp(a):

Protein Pastries! Important Kringles on Lp(a)

Kringle Number	Importance
KIV-2	Dictates production rate of Lp(a). Less KIV-2 repeats = more particle production per unit time
KIV-7 and 8	Site of non-covalent binding of apo(a) to ApoB
KIV-9	Site of covalent (strong) bond of apo(a) to ApoB
KIV-10	Carries oxidized phospholipids

8. **So how do we get rid of it?**
   a. Well, this would mean we would have to know how it's cleared from the body, which we don't. But it's

apparently not cleared by the LDL receptor like the other criminals.

9. **How do you know it's not cleared by the LDL receptor?**
   a. Statins, which work by increasing LDL receptors, actually increase Lp(a), on average, by 19.3%. Statins increase PCSK9 levels, and PCSK9 is involved in Lp(a) production, so this may be one of the reasons for this increase. And in a meta-analysis of statin trials, those with Lp(a) levels above 50 mg/dL NOT on a statin had a 31% increased risk of having a CV event...while those TAKING a statin had a 43% increased risk. Bummer.
10. **So does that mean I shouldn't take a statin if I have high Lp(a)?**
    a. The interpretation is that if Lp(a) is part of your problem, the statin won't help that issue. Statins will reduce the other criminals in your lipid neighborhood, and that's what they claim to do. However, if someone gets a less-than-expected LDL-c reduction from a statin, it's often because that person has high Lp(a).
11. **I heard my cardiologist say that there's an "LDL offset" so that if I lower my LDL enough then I'll be fine.**
    a. You can lower your LDL-c all you want, but INDEPENDENT RISK FACTOR means that regardless of the presence or lack of the other criminals in your neighborhood, you still could have issues with these Lp(a) "felons." This LDL offset philosophy is like telling a person with diabetes who is also a smoker that if they stop smoking, then we can stop worrying about all the risk factors conferred by diabetes. Sure, stop smoking, but that doesn't

magically make the problems of diabetes vanish into thin air.

12. **How do I know if my Lp(a) is elevated?**
    a. CHECK IT. The recommendation right now is to check Lp(a) AT LEAST ONCE in your lifetime. If it's low, you never have to check it again. If it's high, then you know.
13. **Why "at least once" in a lifetime?**
    a. There are certain situations in which Lp(a) can rise and take someone from "borderline high" to "elevated." Menopause is unfair for many reasons, and that is one situation in which Lp(a) levels can rise quite a bit (since estrogen suppresses your true Lp(a) production rate). Statins usually don't increase Lp(a) that much, but they sometimes can cause it to skyrocket, so it's reasonable after starting a statin to re-check as well.
14. **Is there any hope?**
    a. There's ALWAYS hope. There are multiple drugs in development specifically for lowering Lp(a) since we now recognize Lp(a) as an independent risk factor. Since we don't know how it's cleared, but we do know it's produced by the liver, the common approach is to "shut off the faucet in the liver" in regards to Lp(a) production. This is achieved by approaches called anti-sense oligonucleotide (ASO) or small-interfering RNA (siRNA) therapy, which both utilize n-acetylgalactosamine (GalNAc).
15. **You just blew my mind with those words... English, please.**
    a. Basically, GalNAc is an access code unique to the liver so the drug can go in and exert its effects without getting into other organs. Then, once it's in the liver, instead of allowing the complementary strands to "get married" to create the mature Lp(a)

protein, it creates a "disastrous couple" that you know will never work out...think Britney Spears and Kevin Federline. And that "marriage" is quickly annulled so the protein is never produced.

16. **But what about now?**
    a. Well, it becomes an art-of-medicine situation, as there are no medications approved for Lp(a) lowering; the only current approved treatment is *lipoprotein apheresis*, which is a cumbersome process that is essentially dialysis of your lipoproteins. Ezetimibe doesn't do anything to Lp(a) levels. Niacin lowers Lp(a) somewhat, although it also can increase insulin resistance and uric acid. Some people take baby aspirin based on MESA data, the ASPREE trial and Women's Health studies. Testosterone injections reduce Lp(a) modestly, but I seriously doubt that's the reason anyone is using to justify getting on the sauce. But if you have high Lp(a), "not knowing doesn't make it go away," and knowing there are ways to potentially treat it with nuance coupled with the understanding that there are more specific therapies on the horizon should give you reason for hope!

One of my best friends is a great example of how nefarious Lp(a) can be, even in those with optimal Home Security Systems. I helped him qualify for the Boston Marathon, he lifts weights regularly, and he pretty much looks like he just descended from Mount Olympus. His bloodwork showed no signs of insulin resistance, his inflammatory markers were undetectable, and his blood pressure was pristine. His LDL-c was just a shade over 100 and his 10-year risk calculator (which to me is just an excuse for clinicians to plug in numbers, avoid thinking, and pat themselves on the back while probably missing a ton of people with heart disease) was 2.3%. "Keep up the good work, and we'll see you next year," right?!

Although I can be super exhausting as a running partner since I never stop talking, my various musings about lipids encouraged him to tell me about his own family history...which was pretty disastrous. And I kept urging him to get his Lp(a) checked as well as obtain a CAC (remember that Coronary Artery Calcium scan, the colonoscopy of the heart)? He finally got his Lp(a) checked: it was 128 mg/dL (anything over 50 is quite high). Your standard lipid panel will NEVER capture Lp(a)...you have to check it separately. And his CAC? 2814...for reference, any score above zero means you have coronary disease...and those with scores of 300 or higher have equal risk of heart attacks EVEN OVER THE SHORT TERM as those who have had prior cardiac events.

My friend had such extensive heart disease that he had to have open-heart surgery...a 5-vessel coronary artery bypass graft (CABG). And guess what? He's doing amazing, we're still running together, and I get to not only share his story, but continue to enjoy the invaluable blessing of his friendship. And unlike that ridiculous fabricated vignette about my Uncle Rex, this is among the many REAL reasons why I have such a passion for prevention. If I were only relying on 10-year risk calculators, I would have one less priceless gift in my life in addition to countless "what ifs."

Check Lp(a). Just Do It.

Lp(UPDATE):

5:32:04.

1 year ago my friend had open-heart surgery. And one year later, he not only finished the Boise Ironman Triathlon 70.3, he CRUSHED it in a time of 5:32:04.

1 hour for every bypass, and 1 more inspirational chapter in a story that, thankfully, is far from over. And hopefully his story

will continue to inspire thousands more to check Lp(a), obtain CACs, and shift the paradigm from reactionary to PREVENTIVE when it comes to cardiovascular disease!

The word "inspirational" is often overused, but it definitely applies to this situation. He may have picked the wrong parents, but by the grace of God I think we both picked the right friends.

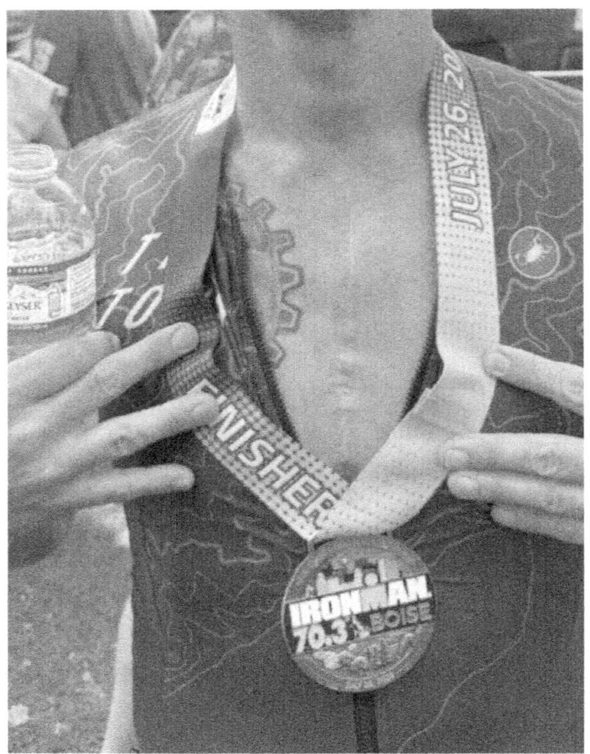

7

UNDERSTANDING YOUR CHOLESTEROL PANEL

"Well, your LDL is a little high but your ratio and your 10-year risk calculator look good, so if you want a flu shot Bonnie will come in here in a minute but otherwise, I'll see you next year!"

-Pretty much every annual wellness visit until someone has a heart attack or stroke

I think there was probably a little too much "king walking" and not enough "common touch" in the last few sections, so let's start off by discussing the components of the lipid panel, which is probably something we all have had checked by our primary care provider. And remember, what we see on a lipid panel is only a small fraction (around 10%) of our total body cholesterol, since all our nucleated cells are producing their own supply. Here are the usual components of a fasting lipid panel:

- **Total cholesterol (directly measured)**
  - But not directly related to cardiovascular risk.
- **HDL cholesterol (directly measured)**
  - And, as we've stated, a plasma measurement of HDL-c gives us NO IDEA of its functionality.

- **Triglycerides (the glycerol component is directly measured)**
    - In general, elevated triglycerides mean insulin resistance, but people can be insulin resistant even with normal fasting trigs. Triglycerides are the component of a fasting lipid panel that is subject to the greatest variation if someone ISN'T fasting (on average ~40% higher in a non-fasting sample).
    - What are "normal triglycerides," you ask? Well, your Lipid Panel will tell you <150 mg/dL, but you probably ought to shoot for <100 since that's where cardiovascular risk REALLY starts to increase. Additionally, 150 is about the 75th percentile of the population...you're only better off than about 1 in 4 people, and we know that 1 in 3 deaths have a cardiovascular cause. So although <150 might work to get a Breakfast of Champions award, I think it's preferable to set the bar a little higher by striving for lower trig levels.
- **VLDL cholesterol (calculated)**
    - Calculated by triglycerides divided by 5...which was the normal ratio of triglycerides to cholesteryl ester on a regular VLDL particle...a normal VLDL particle, that is, in a 1970s U.S. citizen who was probably metabolically healthier than your average standard American in 2024.
- **LDL cholesterol (calculated)**
    - A poor man's estimate of LDL particle count, although there can be significant discordance (a mismatch) between LDL-c and LDL-p. If there are a bunch of little LDL particles carrying scant amounts of cholesterol, you've got much greater risk than your LDL-c would indicate.
- **Non-HDL cholesterol (calculated)**

  - This is simply ascertained by adding up the calculated LDL-c and VLDL-c.
- **Cholesterol/HDL ratio**
  - Ratios are lame and often lead to irresponsible generalizations and misinterpretations...ignore this. Understanding the absolute value of each individual component on the lipid panel is what really matters.

You'll notice that only 3 of the components are actually measured, and then the VLDL and LDL-c levels are estimated. Given that these are the particles that have an ApoB (B for potentially bad) and really are the only ones that can get into your arterial wall, it ought to be a bit unsettling that we're just guessing. Additionally, we know that all these measurements are the MASS of cholesterol in your blood and doesn't tell us the PARTICLES. And we're also missing a pretty important particle measurement, the Lp(a) "felons" that can really wreak havoc in your arterial wall. Since PARTICLES are the potential CRIMINALS in your neighborhood and lipid-mediated risk is related to number of PARTICLES, there appear to be some pretty serious limitations in our standard lipid panel. Can we do better?

So here are some considerations:

1. **Check an Lp(a)...**and then at least you know if you have potential "felons" lurking in your neighborhood.
   a. Lp(a) particles are in the same density range as LDL particles and are thus counted as such on a standard lipid panel.
   b. Although there is an ApoB-100 on each Lp(a) particle, it's important to still check Lp(a) separately, as the ApoB is not the reason why Lp(a) carries such high risk of atherosclerosis.
2. **Check an ApoB**

a. ApoB is a superior marker of cardiovascular risk in numerous population samples such as the UK Biobank and better predicts risk of cardiovascular events in multiple studies such as CARDIA and INTERHEART. Because there is one ApoB-100 molecule on every VLDL, IDL, LDL, and Lp(a) particle and the molecular weight of ApoB-100 stays consistent at 550 kD, this essentially gives us a PARTICLE measurement. And although LDL-c is typically a hair lower in a non-fasting sample, ApoB doesn't really budge. So regardless of whether or not someone is fasting, an ApoB measurement can still accurately quantify the potentially atherogenic particles.

   i. And, once again, particles = criminals. And number of criminals = risk level in your lipid neighborhood.
   ii. However, ApoB in isolation does not tell the particles' origin story. An ApoB in the context of high triglycerides and elevated non-HDL-c is likely rife with REMNANTS...in fact, studies have shown that those with both an elevated ApoB AND non-HDL-c have an 82% greater risk of experiencing a cardiac event even if their LDL-c is "normal!" But an ApoB that's a little on the high end with a normal Lp(a) and low triglycerides may not be as concerning. The broader context always matters!
   iii. Interestingly, it is believed that William Shakespeare was one of the first to recognize the importance of particle metrics when discussing lipid-mediated risk of cardiovascular disease. Using his character Hamlet's emotional discordance as a powerful illustration of the potential discordance between LDL-c and the

number of particles delivering cholesterol, some historians maintain that the original question famously asked in Act 3 Scene 1 was actually, "To ApoB or not to ApoB?"

3. **Check LDL and VLDL particle counts with advanced lipid testing**
   a. An advanced lipid panel (ascertained by either something called nuclear magnetic resonance, or NMR, or another method called ion mobility) can be particularly insightful in identifying DISCORDANCE between LDL-c and LDL-p. It also gives you VLDL-p, which is useful, although it will be unsurprisingly elevated in people with high triglycerides. Advanced lipid testing also gives you the various sizes of HDL, VLDL, and LDL subfractionations.
   b. There are some general associations with VLDL and HDL size subfractionations and metabolic health, but making more definitive statements regarding interpretation of VLDL and HDL sizes requires some context. However, an elevated count of small dense LDL particles (sdLDL) and a consistently small LDL size (Pattern B) are almost unequivocally signs of INSULIN RESISTANCE.

Below are the equivalent percentiles of LDL-c, non-HDL-c, ApoB, and LDL-p.

Table 2: Population Percentiles of Patients Not on Cholesterol-Lowering Medication

Percentile	LDL-c (mg/dL)	Non-HDL-c (mg/dL)	ApoB (mg/dL)	LDL-p (nmol/L) from MESA
5	63	79	54	770
10	72	88	61	870
20	85	103	70	1000
50	112	135	90	1280
70	131	156	104	1480
90	161	191	125	1790
95	176	208	137	1980

| NHANES Data 2005-2016 and MESA LDL-p data 2000-2002

So when LDL-c and LDL-p or ApoB are all similar in regards to percentile, the results are CONCORDANT and the advanced metrics really aren't incredibly useful. But, more often than not, there will be DISCORDANCE between LDL-c and LDL-p, in which case LIPID-MEDIATED RISK FOLLOWS THE PARTICLE COUNT.

A Case Study in Discordance

My wife, who is an absolutely gorgeous, hilarious, brilliant, half-Sicilian half-Puerto Rican (Italurican) spitfire, is a good example of how advanced lipid testing can be useful in early identification of insulin resistance with discordant LDL-c and LDL-p metrics.

She was looking stunning, as always, but was feeling lethargic and lacked subjective mental clarity. So we got some bloodwork, and the pertinent labs are listed below:

- HbA1c: 5.1
- Fasting insulin: 4.8
- Fasting glucose: 80
- Calculated HOMA-IR: 0.95 (<2 is good, <1 is ideal)
- LDL-c: 85 (somewhere between 15 and 20th percentile)

- LDL-p: 1310 (between 50th and 60th percentile)
- sdLDL-p: 545 (elevated)
- Lp(a): 21 nmol/L (never have to check that again, will always be low)

So, here we have a good example of someone who even had normal parameters of glucose metabolism (normal HbA1c, optimal fasting insulin/glucose, sparkling HOMA-IR) and a normal LDL-c BUT significant DISCORDANCE between LDL-c and LDL-p. Additionally, even though we wouldn't think she was insulin resistant by HOMA-IR (and especially not by looking at her), her elevated sdLDL-p demonstrated that she was, in fact, displaying early signs of insulin resistance!

We know from Dr. Gerald Shulman's elegant work at Yale that insulin resistance begins in SKELETAL MUSCLE, and my wife was not exercising at the time she got this bloodwork. So she started going to the gym 2-3x/week and performing a combination of resistance exercise and aerobic work. Nothing monastic or hardcore, just consistent. And she really didn't alter her diet at all, which wasn't super terrible, but still included more Dino chicken nuggets and ice cream than I would personally endorse. And after 3 months, we repeated the labs and here's what we found:

- Fasting insulin/glucose and HOMA-IR were virtually unchanged.
- LDL-c actually went UP to 91 (right around 20th percentile)
- LDL-p: Dropped from 1310 to 994 (just a hair below 20th percentile)
- sdLDL-p: Dropped from 545 to 124 (concordant with other values)

And not only were her labs beautifully concordant, her zest for life had returned, she was cognitively firing on all cylinders again, and she continues to regularly surpass her personal records on both bench press and deadlift. CHA-CHING!

So to summarize:

1. There are limitations in the basic lipid panel, often missing DISCORDANCE between LDL-c and particle metrics, and it cannot identify Lp(a).
2. This discordance can be identified by either getting an ApoB or advanced lipid testing, always viewing each individual biomarker in its broader context.
3. You need to check Lp(a) at least once in a person's lifetime.

Other Advanced Lipid Testing

Some labs, such as Boston Heart Diagnostics, offer testing of ABSORPTION markers as well as PRODUCTION markers. These markers can allow you to operate with some REAL nuance, particularly when selecting lipid-lowering therapies.

- **Cholesterol ABSORPTION markers include CAMPESTEROL and SITOSTEROL**
  - If elevated, this may indicate a benefit for a CHOLESTEROL ABSORPTION INHIBITOR, such as Ezetimibe.
    - Interestingly, carriers of *APOE4* also tend to be hyperabsorbers of cholesterol (more on *APOE4* later in the **Cholesterol in the Brain** section).
- **Cholesterol PRODUCTION markers include LATHOSTEROL and DESMOSTEROL**

- Remember that bifurcated pathway of cholesterol synthesis? Well, these markers can give insight into whether someone is a hyper-producer or under-producer of cholesterol. Interestingly, desmosterol in blood correlates very well with desmosterol in the brain, and low desmosterol is associated with Alzheimer's dementia. Interesting stuff to consider, and we'll discuss that more later.

LDL Triglycerides: The Future of Lipid Metrics?

We've discussed that excess CETP activity results in low HDL cholesterol over time. And this occurs due to heterotypic CETP exchange of triglyceride and cholesteryl ester between ApoB-containing lipoproteins and HDL particles. However, there can also be HOMOTYPIC CETP transfer of triglycerides between different ApoB-containing lipoproteins when triglycerides are chronically and inappropriately elevated. And this can result in excess triglycerides accumulating on LDL particles. Consequently LDL-triglycerides (the triglyceride-richness of LDL particles) has been demonstrated as a risk factor for cardiovascular events in several studies. In fact, those with the highest LDL-triglycerides had a 62% increased risk of heart disease in a recent meta-analysis!

Essentially, the VLDL ApoB-mailmen are incapable of delivering the triglyceride mail because all the mailboxes are full (insulin resistance). So instead, they just give some of their mail to other LDL mailmen who are loitering. Expecting those guys to be responsible and "do another mailman's job" isn't a great idea, and they often end up in the arterial wall.

DEEP DIVE: Advanced Lipid Panels

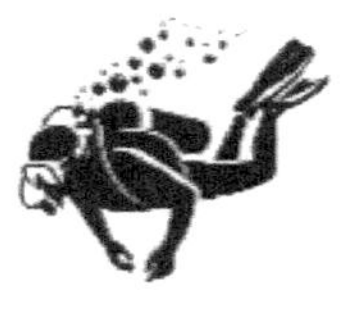

As previously stated, most of the subfractionations of HDL, LDL, and VLDL particles are proxies for INSULIN RESISTANCE. And some labs actually will give you what's called an LP-IR score, which uses the composite data of HDL, LDL, and VLDL subfractionations as a predictor of whether or not someone will eventually develop Type 2 Diabetes. Interestingly, this LP-IR score is actually more predictive of diabetes than more well-known metrics such as HbA1c and even BMI (see, not all risk calculators are garbage)! But before we take the plunge, let these aforementioned core concepts guide our discussion:

1. PARTICLES DICTATE RISK. When ApoB particles are discordantly elevated for a given mass of LDL cholesterol, cardiovascular risk tracks with particle counts.
2. A static measure of HDL-c gives you NO IDEA of its functionality
   a. This also extends to HDL particle quantification and HDL size...although HDL particle counts and sizes may be slightly more correlated with HDL functionality and/or cardiovascular events than HDL-c, it's still reckless to make sweeping generalizations.
3. Advanced lipid metrics as determined by NMR spectroscopy or ion mobility are, in general, additional metrics to identify INSULIN RESISTANCE.

The LP-IR score

The LP-IR score is a composite of 6 different lipid subfractionation measurements. Any score under 30 is ideal, whereas those above 67 (this would be in the top 25%) had a twofold risk of developing T2DM in the Women's Health Study. Similarly, those in the top 25% had a 59% increased risk of diabetes in the MESA cohort. The individual components of the LP-IR score are as follows:

- HDL particles (HDL-p)
- HDL size
- VLDL particles (VLDL-p)
- VLDL size
- LDL particles (LDL-p)
- LDL size

HDL Particles: Quantity and Size

So let's start with our police force, the HDL particles! So, in general, when HDL particles get "fat and fluffy with triglycerides" due to excessive CETP activity, they become like policemen that are TOO BLOATED to pass their fitness test. And then, in the attempted fat loss procedure by unskilled surgeons (hepatic and endothelial lipase), we are left with gaunt, emaciated HDL cops who are now TOO WEAK to pass their fitness test. So the remaining ApoA-1 on the pathetic HDL particles is catabolized by the kidney and eliminated in the urine. This is why we see low HDL-c in people with chronically high triglycerides, and in general this translates to small average HDL particle size and low HDL particle quantity. And in several studies like JUPITER and MRFIT, HDL-p was inversely correlated with cardiovascular events. But, very large (not small) HDL-p was actually associated with INCREASED risk of coronary disease in the EPIC-NORFOLK study...and some of the early studies of fibrates demonstrated that an increase in HDL-p (predominantly of the small variety) was correlated with decreased events! And don't forget, there are between 1 and 5 ApoA-1 molecules on each HDL particle.

And guess what? Both LARGE and SMALL HDL particles have different functions, similar to how large policemen might be better in a fistfight while wiry guys might be able to better run down a fleet felonious fellow. Large HDL particles tend to be better at efficiently delivering their cholesterol cargo via SR-B1 to tissues that may need it, while small HDL particles seem to be more efficient at effluxing cholesterol out of macrophages in the arterial wall...and I'd say both of those functions are pretty important!

(If your brain isn't already resembling a heap of scrambled eggs, there are also different combinations of letters and numbers that are somehow supposed to help us "better define" HDL particle size. For instance, the largest HDL particle is called an HDL-2b particle, whereas the smallest particles are of the HDL-3c variety...and then occasionally people will try to throw some Roman numerals in there. Basically, it makes you want to completely defenestrate alphanumerics and maybe learn something more simple, like Japanese or Arabic).

So if you find this confusing, join the club...there are just too many exceptions and too much conflicting data to use any HDL metric in isolation.

So in summary:

- Small average HDL particles are, in general, associated with INSULIN RESISTANCE.
- Low HDL-p, in general, is associated with INSULIN RESISTANCE
- A static measure of HDL-c (or HDL size or HDL-p) gives you NO IDEA of its functionality.

VLDL Particles: Quantity and Size

VLDL particle subfractionations are quite a bit easier to understand than their HDL counterparts...but then again, so is quantum physics, neurosurgery, and the mystical pleiotropy of Essential Oils (ok, maybe just the first two). In a fasting sample, VLDL particles are the big-time traffickers of triglycerides. And if fasting triglycerides are high, we would expect to see larger quantities of VLDL-p. Hey, that makes sense! And, in general, if there are more triglycerides around (as in insulin resistance), we would expect the average size of these VLDL particles to be LARGER. So, in general, large VLDL-p size is also associated with insulin resistance.

BUT, it couldn't be that easy. Because, despite having a neutral effect on insulin resistance, if someone is taking a PCSK9 inhibitor, it increases the average size of VLDL particles. And additionally, sometimes when a person adopts a low-carbohydrate ketogenic diet, they can also have predominantly large VLDL particles despite having low triglycerides. Darn it! But typically the context will clue you in as to whether or not this may be the case.

So with VLDL:

- Elevated quantities of VLDL-p and large VLDL-p are associated with INSULIN RESISTANCE.
- Large VLDL size is, in general, associated with INSULIN RESISTANCE.

LDL Quantity and Size:

As mentioned, discordantly elevated LDL-p is present in states of insulin resistance because it requires more small particles to transport the same mass of cholesterol. And a small LDL average size (Pattern B for Bad) is almost unequivocally associated with insulin resistance. This shift from Pattern A to Pattern B actually occurs at a fasting triglyceride level of around 95...I told you that a fasting trig of 150 was way too high!

So with LDL-p:

- High quantities of LDL-p, especially when discordantly high for a given mass of cholesterol, are associated with INSULIN RESISTANCE.
- Small average LDL particle size (Pattern B) is almost always associated with INSULIN RESISTANCE.
- And since the NUMBER OF PARTICLES is the NUMBER OF POTENTIAL CRIMINALS in your Lipid Neighborhood, LDL-p gives you a better idea than LDL-c of the type of Lipid Neighborhood you're living in.

Table 3: NMR Values Typically Associated with Non-Insulin Resistant Persons (target values are either below or above the 50th percentile using data from the LipoScience population)

Lipoprotein Metric	Target Value
Small LDL-p	<527 nmol/L
LDL size	>20.8 nm
Large VLDL-p	<2.7 nmol/L
VLDL size	<46.8 nm
Large HDL-p	>4.8 µmol/L
HDL size	>9.2 nm

And now hopefully the waters of Advanced Lipid Testing are just a bit less murky...except, of course, for the HDL section of the pool...that's like the old abandoned hot tub that still harbors a few inches of tepid, stagnant water from Uncle Jay's pool party back in 1994. It's a surefire recipe for cellulitis if you marinate in there too long. So just wade around in the ApoB side of the pool and you'll be fine!

Legs to Die For? Or Legs that Tell Us You're Dying?

Summer is my favorite time of year. With warmer weather comes baseball, backyard barbecues, and a fresh opportunity to identify people with peripheral artery disease (PAD) now that everyone is wearing shorts. Those hairless, rust-colored legs probably won't go far before the calves start crampin', and those folks certainly need to move to a much safer Lipid Neighborhood given their high risk of experiencing major adverse cardiovascular events.

And then sometimes you'll see a person with abnormally chiseled calves; this individual's gastrocnemii would make even the most shredded of bodybuilding bros quite envious. But as your gaze drifts upward, you observe a disproportionately doughy torso. This person likely has some degree of lipodystrophy; he or she has very little subcutaneous fat and any excess adipose quickly spills over into visceral and ectopic depots. Unfortunately, these folks often have severe insulin resistance and significantly elevated triglycerides to accompany those killer legs.

Other Risk Factors to Consider

Obviously, I think 10-year risk calculators or any other calculators where you simply plug in numbers are lame. I think understanding the INDIVIDUAL components included in each risk calculator is far more important than the composite score that some algorithm vomits onto your computer screen. But there are a few more salient risk-enhancing factors that are important to note when determining your INDIVIDUAL risk of cardiovascular disease; these can influence either your Home Security System, Lipid Neighborhood, or both.

- FAMILY HISTORY is a critical factor. As I've said, "picking the right parents" is a big part of this charade. I'm pretty nervous about a person with an Lp(a) of 100 nmol/L who has a horrible family history of premature heart attacks. Conversely, I'm far less uneasy about the person with a potentially worse lab value on paper, but with virtually no cardiovascular events in a family where everyone lives to be 108.

- Certain OBSTETRIC factors such as preeclampsia and gestational diabetes can increase your risk of both cardiovascular disease and diabetes, respectively. Not fair. Early menopause and the general menopausal transition can also affect both the Glucose Homeostasis pillar of your Home Security System as well as your Lipid Neighborhood. Also not fair, but important to recognize.
- As mentioned previously, systemic inflammatory conditions can also predispose you to ASCVD. Certain ethnic groups seem to have outsized predisposition to cardiac disease as well.
- Erectile dysfunction is an early and ominous sign of vascular disease, often preceding cardiac events by 3-5 years. Men with ED have a 25-45% greater chance of experiencing a cardiovascular event, so this "5th Vital Sign" warrants a thorough medical evaluation in our preventive paradigm. If life never gets hard, you need to check your heart.
- Certain conditions like untreated hypothyroidism, biliary obstruction (gallstones), and nephrotic syndrome (frothy, bubbly protein-filled urine), among many others, can lead to secondary causes of elevated cholesterol. It's important to rule those out, particularly if lipid levels were previously normal, but typically other symptoms will lead you down that diagnostic rabbit hole. If you have the energy levels of a comatose walrus, are doubled over in pain after eating an avocado, and need to flush 3 times after peeing, then we may need to check your thyroid, gall bladder, and kidneys, respectively, in the context of elevated cholesterol levels.

In general, however, all the other risk-enhancing factors are either directly or indirectly addressed by the mantra, "Control your insulin, control your life." But now that we have discussed the ways to measure the various elements of our Home Security System and Lipid Neighborhood, we still don't know if any mailmen have gone rogue and crashed into our arterial wall. People don't live on paper, so we are now compelled to ask the question:

Got plaque? Get a CAC!

8

GOT PLAQUE? GET A CAC!

IMAGING FOR IDENTIFICATION OF DISEASE

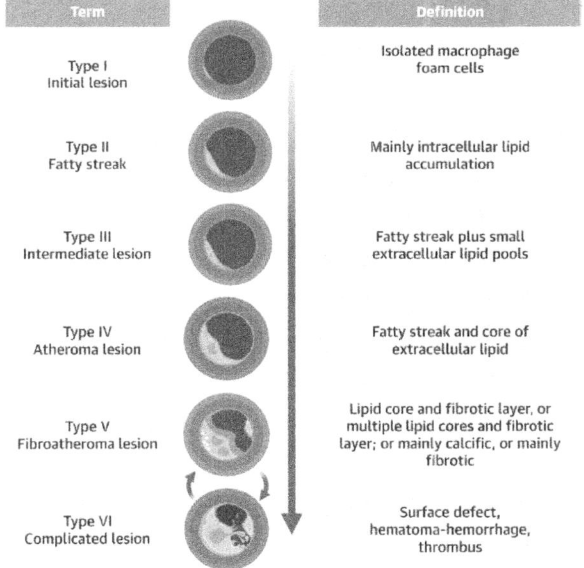

Figure 11: Atherosclerotic plaque progression
Source: Dawson, L. P., Lum, M., Nerleker, N., Nicholls, S. J., & Layland, J. (2022). Coronary atherosclerotic plaque regression: JACC State-of-the-Art Review. *Journal of the American College of Cardiology*, *79*(1), 66–82. https://doi.org/10.1016/j. jacc.2021.10.035

So we've all seen this picture. We know that you cannot have atherosclerosis without a mailman going rogue. But once this ApoB-containing lipoprotein infiltrates the arterial intima, this picture makes it seem like the process of fatty streak/foam cell/fibroatheroma progression slowly and steadily trudges along until a critical degree of STENOSIS, or narrowing, ends up giving you chest pain and occluding your artery. Well, that's NOT how it happens most of the time...in fact, we know from the ICONIC study that 2/3 of heart attacks occur in a vessel with LESS THAN 50% STENOSIS due to rupture of a "vulnerable plaque!" The take-home message is "You're fine...until you're not!"

So, do we have ways of identifying whether or not you've been broken into? We do! And if you HAVE been broken into, we know that there has been a crime scene instigated by an ApoB-containing lipoprotein. We also know the other mailmen are followers by nature and will likely come to the scene of the crime, and well-intending inflammatory citizens will arrive and inevitably make the situation worse...so can we move you to a safer neighborhood with fewer criminals? We can! And various cholesterol-lowering medications have been shown to both stabilize vulnerable plaque and even regress the amount of plaque in your arteries by moving you to a nice, safe gated community where the criminal mailmen won't continue to break in.

So do you "got plaque?" Don't know? Get a CAC!

Coronary Artery Calcium Scans

This "colonoscopy of the heart without the nasty pregame show" is an awesome test for ruling out your risk of having any cardiovascular event AND also gives insight into whether or not you ought to consider taking any cholesterol-lowering medication. Imagine you had a polyp identified during your colonoscopy and the doctor said, "Well, you've got a pre-cancerous growth in your colon. Let's wait around for a few years for you to actually get colon cancer, and then we'll think about treating you." No! You take out the polyp and check back in a few years to repeat the colonoscopy! The same philosophy ought to be applied to heart disease. Waiting around for people with unstable plaque to "have the big one" prior to intervention seems ludicrous, but has been the historical reality of Western Medicine. And this is the paradigm that needs to change!

So we'll discuss the information we can glean from the CAC, highlight the pros of CAC scoring, which are numerous, and acknowledge the limitations, since no test is perfect. Obviously, this entire discussion of diagnostic imaging does not apply to the situation in which you're having crushing chest pain radiating down your left arm...that's exactly what we're trying to PREVENT rather than sitting around waiting to REACT.

When It Comes to CAC, Rewind it Back

Historically, my general approach has been to get your first CAC at age 40, fire up a zero, and then check back in 3-5 years. However, a recent study showed that the mean age of incident CAC in white males was 36...so maybe we ought to consider beginning our preventive screens a bit earlier!

What does the CAC tell me?

The CAC determines if you have calcified plaque in your coronary arteries, which is actually a late finding in the process of atherosclerosis development. Calcified plaque is actually a more stable plaque, meaning less vulnerable to rupture, which is a good thing. But the presence of ANY calcium is evidence there's been a break-in and essentially any residual calcium is a "scab in your arteries." And once you've been broken into, it means that your Home Security System has failed you, and a criminal mailman in your Lipid Neighborhood was able to wreck your arterial wall. Additionally, if your CAC is 300, you have the same

SHORT-TERM risk of having a heart attack as people who have experienced prior myocardial infarctions...yikes!

On the other hand, there is significant POWER OF ZERO with CAC in regards to NEGATIVE PREDICTIVE VALUE, around 99% over 5-15 years. This means that if your CAC score is zero, the likelihood of you having a cardiac event is about as likely as you getting attacked by a pack of wolves. Not very likely.

Got plaque? Get a CAC...and maybe look for TAC, too!

Although having a CAC of zero is generally associated with very low risk of clinical events, people with a high quantity of thoracic aorta calcium (TAC) in the MESA study had a ~80% increased risk of both cardiovascular disease and all-cause mortality...even if their CAC was zero! So looking for "evidence of a break-in" in other arterial beds remains a good idea. TAC can be assessed simultaneously when getting a CAC, but "CACTAC" sounds like the love child of a prickly desert plant and a breath mint, so let's try to maintain our credibility by referring to them separately.

And even if you haven't been particularly diligent about ensuring your Home Security in regards to modifiable risk factors, a CAC of zero still carries a similarly VERY low risk of having an event over 5 years. However, I wouldn't get lulled into a false sense of long-term security. Get your act together now, control your insulin, control your life...but taking any cholesterol-lowering medication probably isn't going to help your cause. A study of over 13,000 patients with a CAC of zero who either took a statin or didn't take a statin were followed for 9.4 years... and the cardiovascular event rate was IDENTICAL. Statisticians like to call this a NUMBER NEEDED TO TREAT, or NNT, which assesses the likelihood that if you gave a bunch of people a medication somebody would actually benefit from it. And the NNT for cholesterol-lowering medication in people with a CAC of zero ranges from 3571 to infinity.

Practical translation from my end? Starting at age 40, get a CAC, fire up a zero, work on your Home Security System, and check back in 3-5 years. Kinda like a colonoscopy, but without the bowel prep and without the unsettling knowledge that someone's head is not up their own backside, but yours. And if you do have a CAC greater than zero, this necessitates a discussion about how to move you from your current criminal-infested neighborhood to a safer gated community using our lipid-lowering toolbox.

Now there are some limitations to CAC, which are listed below:

- Although it's a cheap test, you generally have to pay out-of-pocket, since insurance companies usually won't cover it. Maybe they will read this book and change their policies...
- CAC is not always particularly useful in a younger person. Specifically, if your Home Security System is a disaster and it looks like you live in a rough inner-city Lipid Neighborhood on paper, if you're 35 years old you'll probably still have a score of zero. And a score of zero in that case doesn't confer relative immunity...I'm still nervous about that person, since he may very well have soft, non-calcified plaque due to his risk factors. However, a NON-ZERO score in a young person is meaningful, since from the CARDIA research consortium we know that any score of 1 or greater in a person 32-46 years old carries a 5-fold risk of having a premature event. So you can get a CAC when you're young, but the power of zero just isn't as powerful in that sense; it's actually the power of NON-ZERO that should get you pretty concerned.
- CAC in people with Familial Hypercholesterolemia is controversial, although over ~3.5 year follow-up a CAC of zero even in people with genetically-confirmed FH is

still associated with ZERO events. There are multiple studies showing incredibly low risk in this population when CAC is zero. However, if there is an opportunity to obtain a **CT coronary angiogram (CCTA)** or other modalities such as carotid ultrasound for plaque assessment, it's probably reasonable here, particularly since in the Miami Heart study over a quarter of those with LDL-c >190 had some degree of soft plaque on CCTA, which is a great transition into a brief discussion of that modality.

CT Coronary Angiography (CCTA): CAC on Steroids

CAC is a great test and an awesome screening tool, but CCTA is really the future of imaging. In the past, the ridiculous amount of radiation limited its broader use, but now they have minimized the radiation to 1 millisevert (recall that a CAC has as little as 0.6 msv, which is the same as a mammogram). With CCTA, you not only get to see the calcified plaque, you get to see the following:

- Non-calcified plaque (which includes low-attenuation plaque and other vulnerable features associated with cardiovascular events).
- Degree of stenosis, or narrowing, in each individual coronary vessel.
- Something called fractional flow reserve (FFR) which tells you if blood flow is being restricted.

So CCTA really gives you the best overall picture of the coronary vasculature, and in that Miami Heart Study 13.2% of people with LDL-c <70 had some degree of soft plaque. However, most people with soft plaque either smoke, have diabetes, have hypertension, have high Lp(a), or a combination of these risk factors. Sounds a lot like what we've been discussing this entire time.

Some limitations of CCTA are cost and the need for intravenous contrast, but as far as the information it gives you, it's pretty much the best non-invasive tool we have at this point.

DEEP DIVE: Vulnerable Plaque on the Oregon Trail

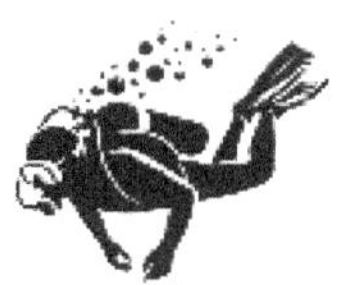

An early Core Memory for children of the late 1980s was playing the Oregon Trail Computer game. You would insert the floppy disk, wait several hours for the computer to boot up, remove the floppy disk after encountering the Blue Screen of Death, blow on the floppy disk, re-insert the disk, and then by the following school day you were ready to play! Even before all of the valuable life lessons gleaned on the trek from Independence, Missouri to the Willamette Valley we were learning PATIENCE and DELAYED GRATIFICATION.

And then we were faced with tough life questions such as the following:

- Should I pack more beef jerky or buy a spare wagon wheel?
- Should I see if I can shoot the agile and elusive squirrels when hunting, or simply wait for the buffalo?
- Should I ford the river or caulk the wagon and float it?
- What is dysentery and why did Jeffrey just die from it?

We were building problem-solving skills, building vocabulary, and unwittingly learning about RESILIENCE. And, quite remarkably, I would sometimes be afflicted with cholera, typhoid fever, a broken leg, and a bad haircut but still survive the journey to the Pacific Coast. But then on other journeys I would only have a mild bout of the flu before the ominous message "Josh has died" would flash across the screen and ruin my day.

And our bodies are really good at NOT DYING; we are masters of Damage Control. And one way that we observe this is something called "Glagovian Remodeling." When a lipoprotein mailman goes rogue into the arterial wall and kicks off the maladaptive immune response that results in plaque formation, the vessel remodels OUTWARD rather than INWARD. Inward remodeling would compromise blood flow, so until a threshold of 40% stenosis is reached, the vessel adapts to preserve the diameter of the vessel.

But, as we know, 2/3 of myocardial infarctions occur in a vessel without any significant degree of stenosis due to a vulnerable plaque rupture. This is because atherosclerosis is a "disease of the donut." Plaque is like mold on a donut; mold is gross, but it takes a lot of mold to encroach into the donut hole. However, that mold can ruin your life at any time if you mistakenly take a bite out of the nasty donut.

So although our bodies are very resilient, identifying any moldy plaque is of paramount importance when discussing prevention of coronary events. Because even a "mild case" of atherosclerosis on paper can lead to a premature end of your proverbial Oregon Trail pilgrimage. Below is a table that shows some of the high-risk plaque features that can be identified with non-invasive imaging and their associations with clinical events.

Table 4: Selected High-Risk Plaque Features and Association with Cardiovascular Events

(Not an exhaustive list by any means...don't hate)

Feature	Description	Risk in Clinical Trials
Low-attenuation plaque (LAP)	<30 HU Appears darker since it absorbs less x-rays due to lipid content	5x risk of MACE when >4% in SCOTHEART
High total plaque burden (TPV)	Commonly used threshold is 238.5 mm3	5x risk of MACE from PROMISE 7x risk of MI from SCOTHEART
Fat-attenuation Index (FAI)	Threshold is <-70.1	4.7x risk of MACE from ORFAN
Non-calcified plaque	"Soft plaque" including fibrofatty and necrotic core	Strongest predictor of MACE in ICONIC
Obstructive Disease	>50% stenosis	Even in 1 vessel obstructive disease, 2.2x risk of MACE from CONFIRM
Multivessel Disease	Risk increases with number of vessels involved	From CONFIRM: 2 vessels: 2.9x 3 vessels: 3.5x 4 vessels: 4.7x

Additional Non-invasive Imaging Tests For Consideration

Briefly, we know that from the PESA study that 44% of the time atherosclerosis starts in the iliofemoral arteries (big arteries coming from your thigh and branching into your lower leg), so some preventive cardiology practices do perform iliofemoral ultrasounds to detect early atherosclerosis. And in PESA, 31% of the time carotid plaque was present even when coronary plaque was absent, so in that case, something called carotid intimal medial thickness (cIMT) with plaque assessment can be helpful.

It's important to not JUST rely on cIMT but also employ the B-mode carotid ultrasound, which allows you to visualize the arterial wall as well as vascular flow. (Blood flow traditionally can be assessed with a different ultrasound called a Doppler). The high degree of variability between sonographers as well as broad population variability in carotid wall thickness has limited this test's utility on a large scale. But if you can find a competent sonographer who performs plaque assessment, this can also help you take a proactive approach to atherosclerosis identification.

Additionally, it may be possible to reverse the progression of atherosclerosis with aggressive lifestyle measures if non-coronary plaque is identified early with these ultrasonographic modalities. Quite encouragingly, 8% of people in PESA were able to achieve plaque regression by really getting their acts together from a lifestyle perspective! Once again, the key point is that we have tools in the toolbox to identify disease in its infancy and intervene accordingly.

A Brief Word About Functional Testing Brought to You By The 42nd U.S. President

"I Did Not Fail My Cardiac Stress Test, Not a Single Time, Never. Those Allegations are False."

When I mention former President Bill Clinton, I know EXACTLY what first comes to your mind. At this point it's almost infamous, but, quite shamefully, he had NORMAL CARDIAC STRESS TESTS every year before finally getting some imaging that revealed that he needed a quadruple bypass surgery. And this parallels what was observed in the PROMISE trial that compared anatomical testing with functional testing.

(Functional tests include stress electrocardiography, stress echocardiography, and nuclear stress testing). 57% of participants in the functional testing group who had cardiovascular events in PROMISE also had NORMAL FUNCTIONAL TESTS.

Go ahead and get a stress test...it's particularly fun to try to "Beat Bruce" (the Bruce Protocol is the name of the treadmill stress test). But a normal stress test doesn't necessarily rule out the presence of coronary disease. So make sure you take advantage of the many non-invasive imaging tests we have that can help us take a preventive approach to cardiovascular disease...I bet President Clinton's ~~intern~~ cardiologist would agree.

So to summarize:

- Got plaque? Get a CAC! Fire up a zero at age 40, repeat every 5 years
- A CCTA gives you the most detail, and it can identify soft plaque, vulnerable plaque features, and identify any blood flow restrictions. This is particularly useful in younger populations, populations with more risk factors, and possibly those with FH.
- Atherosclerosis often begins in other arterial distributions, such as the iliofemoral and carotid, so utilization of ultrasonic modalities, if available, can enhance the preventive approach. And you might be able to pass your stress test, but if you've got plaque, good luck fooling a CCTA.

Invasive Imaging

I've mentioned that we have tools in our therapeutic toolbox that can not only stabilize coronary plaque, but can also, over time, lead to plaque regression. And it's nice that, with the use of invasive imaging techniques such as intravascular ultrasound (IVUS) as well as optical coherence tomography (OCT) and near-infrared spectroscopy (NIRS), this has allowed us to observe the effects of medications in the vascular wall. It's one thing to see an ApoB or LDL-c metric "look better on paper," but it's very encouraging when you can actually demonstrate benefits in regards to arterial plaque quantity and composition.

So what we have observed in a meta-analysis of 17 different IVUS studies is that **for every 1% reduction in percent atheroma volume (PAV), which is a measure of plaque quantity, this is associated with a 20% reduction in cardiovascular events**. I call this "The Power of 1," since when you initially hear this number, it sounds pretty trivial. But a 20% reduced risk of heart attack is much more meaningful.

Additionally, OCT and NIRS can give us even more high-resolution insight into vulnerable plaque characteristics, which include the following:

1. **A THIN fibrous cap** (thicker caps are less likely to rupture)
2. **A LOT of LIPIDS** (more fat in the plaque, more likely to crack)
3. **A lot of INFLAMMATORY CELLS** (those plaques are angry)

And in studies of statins, such as REVERSAL and ASTEROID, we see increased plaque stability and, in some people, some plaque regression. And then with PCSK9 inhibitor trials, such as PACMAN-AMI and HUYGENS, we see even **further plaque regression** (around 2% PAV reduction...remember the power of 1)? Additionally, we see increased STABILITY of HIGH-RISK FEATURES. In these studies, we observed **double** the fibrous cap thickening and about a **twofold decrease** in the amount of lipid and inflammatory cells when using the PCSK9 inhibitors compared to statins alone. And these beneficial changes in plaque composition can occur as rapidly as 2-6 weeks after initiation of therapy...why wait to move to a safer neighborhood when you can be there now?

There is another really cool study that shows a high-intensity interval training protocol reduced PAV over 1% as well, and this effect was independent of cholesterol levels...so there are other factors at play. But the point is that we don't have to wait around for your situation to get worse...we can tackle atherosclerosis head-on and potentially reverse the trajectory of the disease!

It's wonderful that these studies have shown us it's possible to reduce the progression of atherosclerosis. But I also think it's nice that you can avoid a catheterization to determine a medication is stabilizing and regressing your plaque. I would also think as a cardiologist it's probably easier to maintain your friendships if you can avoid having to run hoses up people's groins.

To summarize:

- If you have ANY plaque, as identified by CAC or other imaging modalities, do you want that plaque STABLE or UNSTABLE? (Rhetorical question).
- Do we have tools in our therapeutic toolbox that can confer plaque stability? We do!
- Do we have tools in our therapeutic toolbox that can confer further stability AND potentially regress plaque quantity? We do!
- **Do you want to keep living in the same neighborhood in which you've been broken into, or do you want to live in a nice, safe gated community with fewer criminals?**

A QUICK WORD ABOUT GUIDELINES

"The areas of consensus shift unbelievably fast; the bubbles of certainty are constantly exploding."
-Rem Koolhaas

At this point, we've pretty well established our framework for cardiovascular risk stratification. And it makes sense to move to a nice, safe gated community with fewer criminals if you've been broken into. But what does a "safe, gated community" look like as far as cholesterol levels?

Every few years there will be an "Expert Consensus Statement" or "Cholesterol Guidelines" document that is about 700 pages long and filled with indecipherable flow charts and references to a bunch of clinical studies named after physicists that you've never heard of. It can be tough to make practical sense of these documents for both clinicians and patients alike. So I think it's important to understand the WHY behind the numbers and not just simply treat a cholesterol metric to a certain number because "consensus says." Sometimes consensus is wrong, and sometimes it's reasonable. But that's why we've spent so much time learning the importance of the individual components of our Home Security System and Lipid Neighborhood along with various ways to identify evidence of disease.

So here's my basic summary of the current Cholesterol Guidelines, which blends the European Guidelines, some of the American consensus statements, and the framework we've discussed so far, and it's an acronym:

"Drive F.A.S.T. on Route 55"

F is for FIND disease, since you can't treat what you don't know. Understand the individual factors that contribute to cardiovascular disease, and utilize our various imaging tools to rule out the presence of vascular pathology.

A is for ATHEROSCLEROSIS, and atherosclerosis is ANY PLAQUE identified on CAC or other imaging modalities. Guidelines will use terms like "Primary Prevention" or "Secondary Prevention" in reference to atherosclerosis, but often will say that someone with a CAC of 800 is still "primary prevention" since he or she hasn't "technically had a heart attack or stroke yet." Then once they "have the big one" only then are they reclassified as "secondary prevention." I believe **ANY EVIDENCE OF PLAQUE is really secondary prevention**! Like I've asked *ad infinitum*, do we want to wait around for you to get worse, or should we be proactive now?

S is for STATINS, which, although they have proven benefit in reducing cardiovascular events in numerous clinical trials, are not a panacea. If the year was 2004, we would be relegated to statin use as the primary agent in our medication armamentarium, but times have changed, and so...

T is for TOOLBOX. There are multiple medications that address different cholesterol pathways available to clinicians now, and though statins can be an effective tool, it's important for us to be knowledgeable and proficient with our full toolbox.

Similar to how hypertension and diabetes can be treated with various strategies addressing multiple pathways, lipids can now be treated similarly if necessary.

And **ROUTE 55** is for the LDL-c threshold of 55 recommended for "very high-risk patients with ASCVD." I think terms like "very high risk" and "high risk" in people with atherosclerosis are sort of strange. If you've been broken into, you should move to a safer neighborhood. And if you're using an LDL-c target of 55, you can use the equivalent non-HDL-c and ApoB targets (found in **Chapter 7, Table 2**) to ensure you're not missing discordance. A good rule of thumb is to just use the same LDL-c target for ApoB (so if LDL-c is <55 ApoB would also be <55) and add 30 to the non-HDL-c target (so <85 in this case) and you'll pretty much be in the same ballpark as the most aggressive guidelines.

Drive **F.A.S.T** on **Route 55**...Find Atherosclerosis, and understand that Statins are just one tool in the therapeutic Toolbox for reducing your risk of heart attacks and strokes. As always, CONTEXT IS CRITICAL when determining the Lipid Neighborhood that is ideal for you. Rather than just pedantically focusing on mere numbers like 55, you and your health care provider ought to carefully consider the robustness of your Home Security System as well as the individual risk factors, both environmental and genetic, that would necessitate a move to a Lipid Neighborhood with fewer potential criminals.

How Low is Too Low?

Certain patients, particularly those on a PCSK9 inhibitor, may get their bloodwork back and nearly have a recurrent cardiac event when they see their LDL-c less than 10 mg/dL. And a lot of times people will stop the medication mainly just because the lab value is shockingly low and, since we know the critical importance of cholesterol for so many functions, it just "seems wrong."

Mendelian Randomization

Mendelian Randomization has been referred to as "Nature's Randomized Controlled Trial." Basically, this technique assesses the relationship between a genetic exposure and an outcome of interest. For example, the relationship between genetic variants resulting in lifetime lower LDL-c and coronary disease has been explored using Mendelian Randomization, and this has become the basis for developing drugs that mimic people who have lived in safer Lipid Neighborhoods across their lifespans. These variants include *HMGCR, NPC1L1, ACLY,* and *PCSK9*.

Many experts in the lipid world will argue for a "physiologic" LDL-c of 22-44 or an ApoB of similar value, since "that's what you're born with." Well, that's not the best argument, since in the Copenhagen Baby Heart Study the infants had ApoB levels of 73 and LDL-c levels of 65 to 80 mg/dL by age 2 months. You may also be born with a blood sugar around 30, and I don't see anyone targeting for "physiologic" blood glucose unless your goal is to be in a hypoglycemic coma.

However, if done responsibly in a way that ENHANCES CLEARANCE, it is safe to have very low LDL-c levels. Remember, what we see on a blood cholesterol panel is only about 10% of total body cholesterol. And yes, people who are born with the inability to synthesize cholesterol, a condition called abetalipoproteinemia, have severe neurologic issues, horrible gastrointestinal symptoms, and premature death if untreated. But people born without hardly any PCSK9 (that protein that puts your LDL receptor claw grabbers out of order) live normal lives and just don't get heart disease since they are simply very efficient at CLEARANCE of LIPOPROTEINS. And even if they're having a particularly bad day and going into septic shock, HDL is the primary lipoprotein that delivers cholesterol to the adrenal glands when a little more is needed for corticosteroid synthesis. So they end up being ok. In fact, people lacking PCSK9 seem to die less frequently if they end up in septic shock, although avoiding situations of sepsis is quite preferable. Their mailmen just all go home at the end of the day to the liver. And certain people who have had LDL-c levels <10 on the PCSK9 inhibitor evolocumab for nearly the past decade haven't had any issues except 43% less heart attacks than those with levels >100. So, as always, context matters, and it matters HOW you lower LDL cholesterol if that's the goal...more on this in Chapter 2 of the Deep End of the Community Pool.

And that brings us to a discussion of the lipid-lowering Tools in our Therapeutic Toolbox.

9

THE TOOLS IN THE LIPID-LOWERING TOOLBOX

"It is not the critic who counts, not the man who points out how the strong man stumbled or where the doer of deeds could have done better. The credit belongs to the man who is actually in the arena whose face is marred by dust, sweat, and blood, who strives valiantly... who at the worst if he fails at least fails while daring greatly."
-Theodore Roosevelt

Since I already made the Disclaimer that "Nothing I say is Medical Advice," I feel I'm immune to the lawsuits that would inevitably result if anyone tries the "Kipchoge Challenge" that I'm about to describe.

Most treadmills at your local gym only go up to 12 mph, which is a 5-minute mile. That's pretty quick for your average person, but it's a mere warmup for elite athletes like Eliud Kipchoge, who famously ran the first sub-2 hour marathon with the aid of super shoes on a course with pristine pacing. But if you can find a treadmill that goes 13.1 mph, which is 4:34 mile pace, see how long you can hang. THAT'S THE PACE THAT KIPCHOGE RAN FOR 26.2 miles...you probably can't even make it 0.2, quite honestly, and that's not a personal slight. It's reality.

And there were criticisms about both the environment (perfect pacing) and the equipment (customized carbon-fiber shoes) that enabled Kipchoge to pull of this otherworldly feat. But guess what? HE STILL RAN THE FULL DISTANCE OF A MARATHON IN UNDER 2 HOURS.

Similarly, people often criticize both drug trials and people who employ pharmacological treatments to either improve their Home Security Systems or move to safer Lipid Neighborhoods. They will say things like, "Oh, that person lost weight and got healthy, but they had to use Ozempic." Good for them! They still lost the weight and got healthy...they just used a potent tool in the available toolbox to catalyze the process. And guess what? Life is a MARATHON, not a sprint, and if you are in need of some proverbial Super Shoes to run your best in Life's Marathon, your time still counts. And it may even improve the time you've been allotted in the process when it comes to quality of life.

Additionally, one of the limitations of cardiovascular clinical trials is that when a pre-specified number of clinical events (like heart attacks or strokes) are reached, the trial terminates. Consequently, the trial treats all participants, whether they were in the treatment group or the placebo group, like they died the moment the trial ended, which doesn't give a realistic view of Life's Marathon. This becomes particularly relevant if the person would have otherwise dropped out of the proverbial race without the pharmacologic "Super Shoes" given to them in the trial.

Now don't get me wrong...not everyone needs medications to minimize cardiovascular risk across the lifespan. If you picked the right parents and pull the right levers from a lifestyle perspective, then you may very well be able to run your life's race without the assistance of any prescription medications. But please don't look down on people who may benefit from one of the many tools in our therapeutic toolbox that have proven effective at reducing heart attacks and strokes. Possessing an understanding of how these tools work and who might benefit is a key to effective preventive cardiology practice.

For this section, we are only going to focus on the cholesterol-lowering medications that have shown, in clinical trials, to reduce cardiovascular events (sorry, niacin). I've been in the arena, and I've prescribed ALL of the medications that we are about to discuss. It's a challenge to offer transcendent individual care for patients, particularly when the system often tries to drag you down into a morass of mediocrity, but people are worth the fight. So when we're considering the various tools in our lipid-lowering toolbox, we have to be honest about the following questions:

1. How does the tool work?
2. What are the POSITIVE BENEFITS of the tool?
3. What are the DISADVANTAGES of the too?

And then, if we're really serious about employing a specific tool or tools, we can also ask the following:

4. How does the tool work when USED WITH OTHER TOOLS?
5. Whatever tools or combination of tools I'm using, are the tools COMPROMISING MY HOME SECURITY SYSTEM?

Now before we start a more thorough exploration of the entire toolbox, I want to refer you back to our lipoprotein mailman metaphor to describe the 3 basic medication strategies that address the presence of a corrupt workforce:

1. We can **REDUCE THE NUMBER OF MAILMEN** in the workforce with a **statin** by inhibiting cholesterol synthesis.
2. We can **REDUCE THE AMOUNT OF SPAM MAIL** that you would get in your mailbox that you're just going to discard anyway...so less mailmen end up delivering the junk mail. That's **ezetimibe** and its inhibition of cholesterol absorption.
3. Or, we can just ensure that **ALL THE MAILMEN GO HOME TO THE LIVER AT THE END OF THE DAY,** enhancing lipoprotein clearance with a **PCSK9 inhibitor.**

So let's dive in, starting by paying our respects to a couple of drug classes that are seldom used anymore, at least for the Lipid Neighborhood.

Cholestyramine

1. **How does it work?**
   a. Cholestyramine is a BILE ACID SEQUESTRANT. We know that cholesterol is an essential component of bile, and most bile is reabsorbed from a part of your intestine called the terminal ileum. So if you can't reuse the bile, your liver has to use more of its cholesterol to make more bile, and you'll have less LDL-c in your blood.
2. **What are the positive benefits?**
   a. Cholestyramine did reduce cardiovascular events in an extensive trial a long time ago called the LRC-CPPT and it lowers LDL-c about 20%. Another medication in the class called colesevelam can be used safely during pregnancy.
3. **What are the disadvantages of the tool?**

   a. It interferes with the absorption of a bunch of other medications and is taken as a nasty dissolvable packet several times a day. It also leads to horrible constipation and can elevate your triglyceride levels.
4. **The Verdict**
   a. If somebody has chronic diarrhea maybe they can benefit from off-label use for those symptoms...for lipid-lowering, it's mainly a historical artifact at this point.

Fibrates (Gemfibrozil and Fenofibrate)

1. **How do they work?**
   a. Fibrates are a class of medications called peroxisome proliferator-activated receptor alpha (PPARα) agonists. Basically, they make your liver use fat as fuel rather than producing a ton of triglycerides.
2. **What are the positive benefits?**
   a. Prior to statins, Gemfibrozil did reduce cardiovascular events in the Helsinki Heart Trial and another one called VA-HIT. It reduces triglycerides, which can be helpful if risk of pancreatitis is high, and it does seem to prevent progression of diabetic retinopathy. In some people it can lead to a nice reduction in LDL particle counts.
3. **What are the disadvantages of the tool?**
   a. If used with statins, Gemfibrozil can cause rhabdomyolysis, which is when your muscles end up undergoing mass destruction and you start peeing out what looks like cherry cola...I've had rhabdo on a number of occasions and it can be life- threatening (not from fibrates or statins...long story). Fenofibrate can be used with a statin, but didn't reduce cardiovascular events in studies like FIELD and

ACCORD. And another fibrate, Pemafibrate, disappointingly failed to reduce cardiac events in the more recent PROMINENT trial as well.

4. **The Verdict**
   a. Fibrates are an interesting drug class, and in certain people may be helpful in reducing LDL particle counts. At this point, a fibrate is probably best suited to reduce pancreatitis risk by reducing triglycerides and may prevent retinopathy progression in those with diabetes.

Statins

Ok, deep breath...perhaps no topic is as controversial or contentious as the discussion of statins. Some people think our crops should be sprayed with an Atorvastatin aerosol, while others are certain that tsunamis, forest fires, moral impropriety, and all existential angst is directly related to statin prescription. So here we go!

1. **How do they work?**
   a. Statins inhibit HMG-CoA reductase, which inhibits cholesterol synthesis. My buddy Ryan, who is a fantastic physician, likes to say they "choke the liver out of cholesterol," which in turn makes more LDL receptors (the claw grabbers) go to the cell surface and pull more cholesterol into the cell. Referring back to our lipoprotein mailmen metaphor, they reduce the work force.
2. **What are the positive benefits?**
   a. Statins have more data than any drug in regards to reducing cardiovascular events, and it's not even close. From the 4S trial in 1994 to WOSCOPS to JUPITER and many others, the clinical trial data is immense.

b. Moderate doses of statins reduce LDL-c 30-50%, while high-intensity statins reduce LDL-c around 50% or maybe a bit more. And they do reduce hs-CRP levels.
c. Studies such as REVERSAL, ASTEROID, and SATURN demonstrate increased coronary plaque stabilization effects.

3. **What are the disadvantages?**
    a. The side effects of statins are DOSE-DEPENDENT, meaning that as you increase the dose, you increase the risk of problems. And although almost every side effect under the sun has, at some point, been attributed to statins, we are going to focus on the Big 3:
        i. Muscle pains (a real effect)
            1. Although in many studies patients on statins have also reported similar muscle symptoms on the placebo, statins do inhibit complexes III and IV of the electron transport chain in skeletal muscle mitochondria. This leads to a reduction in oxidative phosphorylation by over 30% EVEN IN ASYMPTOMATIC PEOPLE. Translation: your battery doesn't get charged to full capacity in your muscles if you're on a statin. There's a reason why pro athletes can rarely tolerate any dose of statin, and there are other mechanisms involving calcium handling that contribute to the myopathic effect. However, if you've been recommended a statin, chances are you didn't just qualify for the CrossFit Games or the Tour de France...those guys tend to be interested in other types of "pharmaceuticals."

   ii. In animal studies, regular exercise prior to initiation of a statin does partially attenuate statin-associated myopathy. However, I doubt that these rats performed Google searches on statins prior to taking their Lipitor, so whether or not this translates to humans is unclear. Although exercise is always the answer and almost certainly would help attenuate any perturbations in glucose metabolism while on a statin, if the statin is impairing exercise tolerance then it would certainly be reasonable to consider combination or alternative approaches to lipid-lowering therapy.

b. New-onset diabetes/worsening of blood sugars (a real effect)
   i. A recent meta-analysis of well over 100,000 patients showed that with a moderate dosage of statin, there was a 10% increase in new- onset diabetes over 5 years. And with high- intensity statins, a 36% increase! That's certainly not trivial, and although there are multiple mechanisms for this effect (including reduction of GLP-1 and increased PCSK9), the most clear-cut, in my opinion, involves something called geranylgeranylpyrophosphate, or GGPP. This is an important intermediate in the cholesterol synthesis pathway, and the end result of GGPP production is GLUT4 translocation to the muscle cell surface. However, if you inhibit cholesterol production with a statin, you also inhibit GGPP production. Less GGPP, less GLUT4, less glucose in the muscle...and that's why we see muscle insulin resistance and elevated blood sugars. But, once again, these side effects are dose-dependent.

ii. Dementia (at the population level, no harm).
    1. Lipids in the brain are a complicated topic. In contrast to ezetimibe and the PCSK9 inhibitors, all statins cross the blood brain barrier, and it's likely that many people derive a net benefit from statins in regards to various dementia types. Conversely, it's possible that certain people in which cholesterol synthesis is over-suppressed, perhaps identified by low desmosterol, may experience some negative effects. But this remains in the theoretical realm...certainly more to learn, and this is my personal area of ongoing research.

4. **The Verdict**
   a. Statins do a lot of good things, and the things that we don't love about them increase when the dose increases. Given that most of the initial benefit is from the first dose and each subsequent doubling of the statin only lowers LDL-c another 6%, it makes sense to use statins in combination therapy with other agents to minimize the DOSE-DEPENDENT SIDE EFFECTS. Because the best medication, if there's a reason to take it, is the one that you will keep taking AND will minimize any damage to your Home Security System. And even from a clinical trial standpoint, there isn't much of a compelling reason outside of acute coronary events to reach for the King Kong statin dose.
   b. Combination therapy also makes a ton of sense if we understand cholesterol homeostatic pathways. Basically, your body IS FIGHTING YOU to remain in that SAME ROUGH NEIGHBORHOOD where there's been a break-in. Here's what I mean:

        i. When you inhibit cholesterol synthesis with a statin, your body INCREASES ABSORPTION.
            1. So consider adding ezetimibe to your statin... 2 pathways, better tolerability, more LDL-c reduction...and this approach has been validated in clinical trials such as RACING.
        ii. And statins INCREASE PCSK9, which we know puts your LDLr claw grabbers out of commission. Once again, your body is fighting you!
            1. So statins and PCSK9 inhibitors work quite well together also, and we know that the combination of those two can further benefit coronary plaque and reduce cardiovascular events more than the statin can by itself.
    c. One potentially useful agent for combating statin-associated muscle symptoms is creatine. Several small studies have demonstrated actual benefit with creatine supplementation, with one recent trial showing a >50% subjective improvement of muscle symptoms in over half of the participants. Mechanistically, since statins inhibit creatine synthesis (via the enzyme guanidinoacetate methyltransferase); creatine supplementation should help restore normal levels. Since there's really no downside, it's worth a shot!

5. **BONUS COVERAGE! Hydrophilic vs. Lipophilic Statins**
    a. Astute readers will recognize that some statins (like Pravastatin and Rosuvastatin) are hydrophilic, while others like Atorvastatin and Simvastatin are lipophilic. Hydrophilic means "water loving," and essentially this characteristic makes the statin more water soluble, whereas the "lipid-loving" quality of lipophilic statins makes them more readily dissolve

in fats. Hydrophilic statins tend to be more selective to the liver, which is the organ that expresses the most LDL receptors, whereas lipophilic statins tend to get into non-hepatic sites more easily, including skeletal muscle.

b. Some studies suggest greater potential for muscular side effects with lipophilic statins, but real-world studies show that both hydrophilic and lipophilic statins can result in muscle symptoms along with perturbations in blood sugar. At the end of the day, understanding the hydrophilicity and lipophilicity of various statins can help a clinician operate with painstaking nuance, but I would encourage us all to be **"combophilic"** above all else. Using a lower dose of a statin in combination with other therapies seems to mitigate any side effects better than merely focusing on the solubility.

Ok, that was *ridiculous*. But here are the key takeaways:

- Statins reduce LDL-c, stabilize plaque, and have a ton of data in reducing cardiac events.
- **The initial dose of the statin gives you the most benefit**...each subsequent doubling doesn't do much for lowering LDL-c, but greatly increases risk of side effects.
- The muscle and blood sugar side effects of statins are legitimate physiologic phenomena.
- Statins increase cholesterol absorption as well as PCSK9 levels, **so using them in combination with other medications involving these pathways can help you move into a safer Lipid Neighborhood while minimizing damage to the Home Security System.** Your body fights you tooth-and nail to remain in the same neighborhood in which there's been a break-

in, since "this is home!" But if you can use multiple tools in the toolbox, you can overcome this resistance and live happily ever after.

Ezetimibe

1. **How does it work?**
   a. Ezetimibe makes NPC1L1, the "ticket taker to the cholesterol party" in the gut, more discriminate, thus inhibiting cholesterol absorption. It reduces the delivery of spam mail that you'd just throw away, so less mailmen are out in your bloodstream wasting their time delivering it.
2. **What are the benefits?**
   a. By itself, it lowers LDL-c about 20-25%. But it did reduce events when added to a statin in the IMPROVE-IT trial and there is a trial called EWTOPIA in Japan that, by itself, reduced cardiac events by 34%. Additionally, it helps minimize the dose-dependent side effects of statins, as discussed above.
3. **What are the disadvantages?**
   a. Not much...it's pretty well-tolerated in general, but not very potent.
4. **The Verdict**
   a. An underutilized agent that complements other more potent therapies nicely. If cholesterol markers of absorption (campesterol and sitosterol) are elevated, these can identify people who may benefit a little more from ezetimibe.

> **A Trick for Gallstones?**
> In animal studies, ezetimibe helps dissolve gallstones since most gallstones are cholesterol-rich. Additionally, ursodeoxycholic acid (UDCA), a tertiary bile acid, can be prescribed to further reduce the cholesterol saturation of the bile. Taken together, the combination of ezetimibe and UDCA can pharmacologically dissolve gallstones; I successfully used this on several occasions in clinical practice.

Bempedoic acid

1. **How does it work?**
   a. It inhibits something called ATP citrate lyase, which is one step up from HMG-CoA reductase in the cholesterol synthesis pathway, but bempedoic acid is specific to only the liver. This is an incredibly cool drug from a biochem nerd standpoint, but I'll spare you the details of what can happen when you split citrate into oxaloacetate and acetyl-CoA (you're welcome). Essentially, it's like a low-dose statin that doesn't affect blood sugars and doesn't get into your skeletal muscle.
2. **What are the benefits?**
   a. It reduces LDL-c around 18-21% by itself, but it is available in a one-pill combo with ezetimibe, which results in a 38% LDL-c reduction. It reduces hs-CRP around 22%. And it did reduce cardiovascular events in a study of statin-intolerant folks called CLEAR-OUTCOMES.
3. **What are the disadvantages?**
   a. It can raise uric acid levels and there is a very small increase in risk of gallstones, but it's pretty clean.

4. **The Verdict**
    a. Very clever drug, just not very potent. But nice that it doesn't affect blood sugars or muscles.

PCSK9 Inhibitors (both monoclonal antibodies and inclisiran)

1. **How do they work?**
    a. PCSK9 puts the LDLr "claw grabbers" out of order by targeting the LDLr for lysosomal degradation, so inhibiting PCSK9 increases the availability of LDL receptors to enhance clearance.
        i. Monoclonal antibodies are "perfect mops" of 100% of PCSK9 within 4 hours of injection (Think "mop-oclonal" antibody). Inclisiran, as a GalNAc-siRNA, "shuts off the faucet" of PCSK9 production in the liver, where 2/3 of PCSK9 is produced.
2. **What are the benefits?**
    a. Monoclonal antibodies (evolocumab and alirocumab) reduced cardiovascular events in the FOURIER and ODYSSEY trials, stabilize and regress coronary plaque, lower LDL-c ~60%, and lower ApoB ~50%.
    b. Inclisiran does not yet have any cardiovascular outcome data, but reduces LDL-c ~45%.
3. **What are the disadvantages?**
    a. Not much. Occasionally some people get injection site reactions, since these are injections once every 2 weeks.
    b. Inclisiran is less potent mechanistically than the monoclonal antibodies due to inhibiting less PCSK9, but it is dosed once every 6 months as an injection, which may be more convenient for certain individuals.

4. **The Verdict**
   a. Potent and well-tolerated, doesn't affect blood sugars or muscles, but remains underutilized. Evolocumab and alirocumab are preferred at this time due to their long-term safety profile and proven benefits in reducing cardiovascular events.

Icosapent Ethyl (high-dose eicosapentaenoic acid, or EPA)

1. **How does it work?**
   a. Magic! Well, that's not too far from the truth. EPA is an omega-3 fatty acid, and it seems to stabilize cell membranes, reduce oxidation of LDL, and improve the ratios of other fatty acids to confer endothelial benefits. It also decreases the likelihood of cholesterol crystal formation under conditions of high blood sugars. Interestingly, past trials of combination omega-3 products using EPA and DHA (like the STRENGTH trial) did not reduce cardiac events.
2. **What are the advantages?**
   a. It reduces triglycerides, although the cardiovascular outcome benefit in the REDUCE-IT trial was independent of the effect on triglycerides. It also has shown benefit in reducing high-risk coronary plaque characteristics in studies such as EVAPORATE and CHERRY.
3. **What are the disadvantages?**
   a. It carries a small increased risk of atrial fibrillation and bleeding events.
4. **The Verdict**
   a. Current guidelines suggest benefit in people with coronary disease or at high-risk of events whose triglycerides are 135 or above, which is very

reasonable given the somewhat nebulous and diverse mechanisms of action.

Omega-3 Index

A recent meta-analysis estimated that the risk of fatal coronary disease would be reduced by about 30% if someone merely went from an omega-3 index of 4% (pretty low) to >8% (pretty high). Since this is readily measurable and readily actionable, this seems to be another reasonable metric that could motivate you to eat some salmon or find a quality supplement to boost your levels if your omega-3 index is closer to a Nomega-3 one.

DEEP DIVE: CETP Inhibition

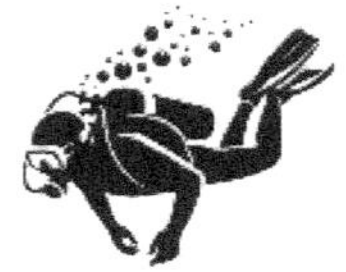

Near the beginning of the 21st century, pharmaceutical companies fell prey to the fallacy that "raising the good cholesterol" must be a good idea, and multiple companies (whom I will not refer to by name just because they get weird about this stuff) attempted to raise HDL via CETP inhibition. If you have less CETP activity, then those HDL particles won't get fat and fluffy with triglycerides and they won't donate their cholesterol to ApoB-containing particles, so HDL-c will increase. And instances in which CETP activity was increased (ahem, insulin resistance) seemed to correlate with increased cardiovascular events, so the thought was that CETP inhibition would be a great way to complement LDL-c reduction to mitigate ASCVD.

The first attempt at this strategy was made by the same company who inadvertently restored the romantic zest in the lives of many couples with a failed blood-pressure drug (rhymes with Niagara). This first CETP inhibitor was called Torcetrapib and the trial was called ILLUMINATE; however, the light was permanently snuffed out for many people in this tragic trial and it was stopped early because people were dying. Unfortunately, some red flags were ignored in the pre-clinical phase of drug development and this drug had off-target effects on the renin-angiotensin-aldosterone system. This led to elevations in blood pressure and also messed up adrenal function; they would've been much better off just giving people more little blue pills.

Still bullish on the strategy of "raising HDL" in efforts to reduce heart attacks, 2 other drugs called Dalcetrapib and Evacetrapib were employed and, although they didn't hurt anyone, these trials were stopped early because they just weren't effective. And then a fourth trial called REVEAL using an agent called Anacetrapib actually worked... sort of.

- REVEAL is still the largest lipid-lowering trial ever conducted, enrolling over 30,000 patients.
- Around the time of REVEAL, people were finally realizing that raising HDL cholesterol pharmacologically just isn't any good; we just can't ensure that these HDL particles will be functional by simply increasing their quantity. However, in looking at folks with genetic loss-of-function in the CETP gene, it was noted that CETP variants that not only raised HDL-c, but also resulted in a lower LDL-c and ApoB, actually had about 16% less coronary events. This was consistent with other genetic variants such as HMGCR and PCSK9.
- So, REVEAL actually reduced the incidence of major adverse cardiovascular events by 9%. However, people in that trial were enrolled with a baseline LDL-c of only 61 mg/dL...and the drug only lowered LDL-c 11 mg/dL. Although that fell in line with what was achieved in other trials of other therapies, it was considered underwhelming and further development was discontinued.

- Additionally, Anacetrapib remained in people's fat cells interminably, which made the manufacturers skittish about continuing to pump a modestly effective drug into people's ample supplies of adipose without knowing the long-term consequences.

So we've all given up on CETP inhibition, right? WRONG! There is a new CETP inhibitor in development called Obicetrapib (since Obi-wan-kenobi was awesome and also since Obi is the Swahili word for heart). This CETP inhibitor not only raises HDL-c (which we don't think really matters), but also lowers LDL-c and ApoB much more than previous iterations. So will the 5th time be the charm for CETP inhibition? That remains to be seen!

Summary

I think a strong case, both biochemically and from clinical trial data, can be made for combination therapy. Addressing multiple pathways with multiple tools employing varied mechanisms of action can help you get into a safer Lipid Neighborhood while minimizing any damage to your Home Security System. The following chart helps summarize the utility and function of some of the aforementioned tools.

Table 5: Selected Lipid-Lowering Therapies

Agent	Mechanism of Action	Translation	Expected LDL-c reduction	Cardiovascular Outcomes
Bile acid sequestrants (Cholestyramine)	Inhibits 7α-hydroxylase, increasing LDLr	Less cholesterol for bile production, so more pulled into the liver	~20%	LRC-CPPT
Fibrates (Gemfibrozil, Fenofibrate)	PPARα agonist, enhances hepatic fatty acid oxidation	Less triglyceride production	~10%	Gemfibrozil: VA-HIT and Helsinki Heart Trial
Statins	Inhibits HMG-CoAr, increasing LDLr	"Cuts the work force" of ApoB mailmen	High-intensity ≥50%	Numerous: 4S, WOSCOPS, JUPITER, many others
Sterol absorption inhibitors (Ezetimibe)	Inhibits NPC1L1 at intestinal brush border and hepatobiliary interface	Decreases the amount of spam mail delivered by the ApoB mailmen that you would just end up chucking	~20-25%	IMPROVE-IT
PCSK9i mAbs (Alirocumab, Evolocumab)	Binds extracellular PCSK9, prevents LDLr degradation	A "perfect mop" of 100% of PCSK9. Makes sure the mailmen return home.	~60%	Alirocumab: ODYSSEY Evolocumab: FOURIER
PCSK9i siRNA (Inclisiran)	Inhibits hepatically produced PCSK9	"Shuts off the faucet" of liver PCSK9 production (2/3 of PCSK9)	~45%	None at this time
Bempedoic acid	Inhibits ATP citrate lyase in liver, decreases synthesis and raises LDLr	Liver-specific "statin" that doesn't get into your muscles or affect blood sugars	~20%	CLEAR-Outcomes

Supplements

Many people prefer a "natural" approach when discussing a potential move to a safer Lipid Neighborhood. Ironically, many of these folks would cheerfully spend $400 a month on supplements rather than even consider a conversation about prescription medication. And just because something is "natural" doesn't mean it's safe or useful...some rather delicious-looking mushrooms were your curious and impulsive cousin Devin's last meal, and they were certainly "natural."

I will always meet people where they're at, but the trouble with supplements is that, other than creatine, they mostly fall into these three basic categories:

1. Possibly useful in the right dose at the right time in the right person.
2. A generally bad idea.
3. Helping to fund your chiropractor's next vacation.

Additionally, many supplements are an unregulated proprietary blend of snake oils, fillers, and traces of lawn clippings that may or may not contain the purported constituents.

I fully intend to write another book on supplements to help folks find the signal amidst the noise in that department, but for now, the table below will hopefully satisfy your yearnings and at least make you think twice prior to consuming expensive, poisonous fungi.

Table 6: Non-exhausting, Non-exhaustive List of Supplements

Supplement	Mechanism/Effects	Comments
Red yeast rice	It's basically unregulated mystery-meat lovastatin at variable and unknown dosages	If you're going to take a statin, I'd advise against a first-generation crappy Costco one
Nattokinase	-Possible inhibition of LDL oxidation along with fibrinolytic effects -15-17% reduction in TG and LDL-c at high doses -May be synergistic with aspirin -Product of fermented soybeans (Effervescent Edamame, perhaps)?	At doses of 10,800 FU in one retrospective study, carotid plaque regression was observed (FU is Fibrinolytic Units, not showing Big Pharma an undignified finger)
Berberine	-Weak PCSK9 inhibitor -Similar to Metformin in AMPK activation	-May lower LDL-c 10-20% along with some benefits in blood glucose
Citrus bergamot	The platypus of cholesterol supplements...purportedly inhibits ACAT and MTP (reduces TG synthesis), activates AMPK, decreases SREBP1-c (increases fatty acid oxidation), indirectly inhibits HMG-CoAr (statin-ish), inhibits NPC1L1 (ezetimibe-esque) increases bile acid synthesis	Highly variable reduction in LDL-c (7-40%) and TG (11-39%)
Plant sterols	Competes for absorption of sterols in the enterocyte, thus reducing LDL-c a little (maybe 10%)	For hyperabsorbers of phytosterols, this could be problematic since they're basically toxic and can also impede absorption of fat-soluble vitamins
Lactobacillus	Converts gut cholesterol to cholestanol, so you poop it out Lowers LDL-c a smidge	Maybe just eat some yogurt

A Word to the Clinicians

Becoming a maestro of medications and a technician of the toolbox is an important component of preventive practice. But oftentimes, the most critical prescription you and I could ever confer is HOPE. No one ever said, "I wish I invested less time in someone I loved." No one ever said, "I wish I had fewer meaningful relationships." No one ever said, "I wish I squandered more opportunities to touch lives." That's why we all got into this in the first place, and it's easy to forget that when you're drowning in a quagmire of prior authorizations and unsigned charts. And learning the best ways to manipulate biochemical pathways for optimization of patient health will help refine your methodological approach and legitimize your clinical acumen. But no one *cares* how much you *know* until they *know* how much you *care*.

PART III

THE ENDOCRINE THERMOSTAT

I've always enjoyed writing papers (shocker), but every now and then in English class we were encouraged to "explore alternative modes of learning." I approached these opportunities with a mixture of disdain and consternation, preferring to simply continue writing my scintillating essays. Given that an unsharpened Number 2 pencil possesses more intrinsic artistic flair than I do, I asked my teacher if I could "perform a song" when assigned a project on Shakespeare's *The Taming of the Shrew*. So I performed a rap entitled, "Whatcha Gonna Do with the Shrew, With the Shrew?" and a hilarious precedent was set for the entire duration of my High School experience. What began as a convenient excuse to avoid pastels and watercolors eventually resulted in my buddy and I forming a hip-hop duo aptly called OTP, short for Overcome the Persecution, which included my friend, Sweet J, and myself, J-Wagz. Sweet J would beatbox at pep assemblies while I would, somewhat disingenuously, rap about the elite talent and transcendent intellect of our student body. I even wore fake stud earrings and a gold chain with a dollar sign roughly the size of my head while we would perform in front of the school. Capitalizing on our popularity, we recorded an album that even featured a special guest, Big Dismal, who laid down some decadently funkalicious basslines on several tracks. (Big Dismal was, in fact, my father, a filial collaboration rarely, if ever, observed within the rapping fraternity). On this controversial album, which is reported to have sold approximately 23 copies worldwide, we addressed difficult topics such as using Rock, Paper, Scissors as an alternative to gang violence and even made a song called G.R.A.D. to commemorate our high school graduation. (G.R.A.D. was a parody of a popular 50 Cent song released around the same time about a less reputable four-letter occupation). And that paved the way for me to progress through academia, become a Lipid Specialist, and write these books that you're hopefully enjoying. Sort of. Maybe. Indirectly.

And the Endocrine System also plays indirect roles in the Home Security System and the Lipid Neighborhood.

The Endocrine System has been referred to as the body's "thermostat" given that the hormonal cascades and their respective feedback loops function similarly to a properly regulated central heating system. And although they may not always directly compromise the Home Security System, dysregulated endocrine factors can make the metabolic milieu less optimal. And when the temperature inside the physiologic abode is "uncomfortable," this can set the stage for a lipid criminal to "break in." So let's discuss some of the hormones that can, usually indirectly, affect an individual's lipid metrics and associated risk factors for atherosclerotic vascular disease.

1

THYROID AND ADRENAL FUNCTION

"Heal your thyroid with this protocol! A daily undrinkable kelp smoothie, weekly chiropractic adjustments, and eating 2 Brazil nuts a day while meditating under a UV lamp, and you'll leave your Hashimoto's in the dust!"

-Every magazine in the Whole Foods checkout line

So why are we discussing the thyroid in a book about cholesterol? Well, as you'll see, since the thyroid gland is sort of the master regulator of just about everything, it also plays a role in cholesterol homeostasis. And although I'm not going to teach you about differentiating between amiodarone-induced thyrotoxicosis Type 1 or 2 or ruminate on the histology of Huerthle Cell Carcinoma (things I did see when I was in practice), I think a basic understanding of thyroid physiology will be helpful given the ubiquity of "thyroid problems" in our society.

1. **What is the basic feedback loop of the Hypothalamic-Pituitary-Thyroid (HPT) axis?**
   a. Similar to most endocrine feedback loops, the hypothalamus releases a releasing hormone, in this case Thyroid Releasing Hormone (TRH). This

signals the anterior pituitary gland to produce Thyroid Stimulating Hormone (TSH), which then instructs the thyroid gland itself to produce the thyroid hormones thyroxine (T_4) and triiodothyronine (T_3). These are called T_4 and T_3 because they are both iodotyrosine molecules with 4 and 3 iodines attached, respectively. In cases of primary hypothyroidism where the thyroid is the culprit, TSH will be HIGH and thyroid hormones will be LOW. In cases of primary hyperthyroidism, TSH will be LOW and thyroid hormones will be HIGH. The pituitary is trying to tell the thyroid to "get with the program" or "slow down, buddy" in conditions of primary hypothyroidism and hyperthyroidism, respectively. But in these cases, the thyroid isn't really listening. Below is a graphic of the basic HPT axis feedback loop:

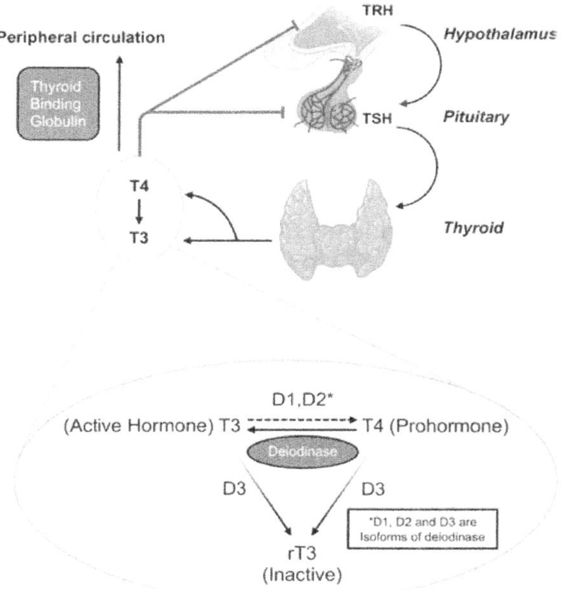

Figure 12: The HPT Axis: The hypothalamus produces TRH, which signals the anterior pituitary to produce TSH, subsequently directing the thyroid gland to produce T4 and T3. If adequate levels of thyroid hormone are produced, TRH and TSH should decrease accordingly. Brown, E. D. L., Obeng-Gyasi, B., Hall, J. E., & Shekhar, S. (2023). The thyroid hormone axis and female reproduction. *International Journal of Molecular Sciences*, *24*(12), 9815. https://doi.org/10.3390/ijms24129815

2. **What is the "recipe" for thyroid hormone synthesis?**
   a. I like to think of thyroid hormone synthesis like baking a batch of chocolate chip cookies...let's just say it's a "Baker's Dozen" in which 12 T4 cookies and 1 special T3 cookie are produced in a batch given the normal physiologic ratio of T4 to T3 production. The special T3 will be quickly "gobbled up" given that T4 is essentially a precursor and T3 is the active thyroid hormone that "makes the magic happen" in

exerting its litany of biological effects. The recipe is quite simple and proceeds like this:

i. Using a thyroid peroxidase (TPO) mixer, incorporate some tyrosine and iodine "chocolate chips" into the thyroglobulin dough, and then distribute the cookies out into the circulation!

ii. The T3 cookie is eaten first, and the T4 cookies are converted to T3 by deiodinases (D1 deiodinase in the liver and D2 elsewhere). If the cookies are left "uneaten," so to speak, thyroxine is converted into something called Reverse T3, or RT3, that has the same quantity of iodines as active T3. However, since the 4th iodine is cleaved from the inner ring rather than the outer ring of the molecule, it is biologically inert.

    1. People with "euthyroid sick syndrome" have normal or low TSH levels but high RT3...this can occur in hospitalized, critically ill patients as your body's way of "delaying death," since it's not in your best interest to rev up your metabolic rate when you're actively dying.

3. **So what sort of symptoms occur in hypothyroidism?**

    a. Pretty much anything you can think of. The classic symptoms are fatigue, weight gain, brain fog, and constipation. And as someone who has had a TSH north of 17 mIU/L (normal is about 1), you can feel pretty bad when your thyroid tanks. Basically, all your metabolic processes screech to a halt and you're the weirdo who is still wearing a hoodie when it's 98 degrees outside. You might be nominally alive, but you're dead on your feet. My resting heart rate was in the high 20s at one point after a spell of thyroiditis, and although I was a very fit endurance athlete, I might as well have been going into hibernation.

Hypothyroidism can also result in acquired von Willebrand Syndrome; interestingly, I had nosebleeds around the clock when I was severely hypothyroid.

4. **And what about hyperthyroidism?**
    a. Quite the opposite...your heart rate is through the roof and you may even go into atrial fibrillation. You're having an internal anxiety attack at all times. You're hot, sweaty, and feel like you've drank a 12 pack of Monster Energy Drinks, and you're generally losing a bunch of weight, but not in a good way. If you want to take a deep dive on Graves' Disease and other causes of hyperthyroidism as well as discuss radioactive iodine, thyroidectomy, and methimazole, I'm sure you can find a riveting Endocrinology textbook to satisfy those yearnings. But I'm not going to cover that here.
5. **What effect does the thyroid have on cholesterol levels?**
    a. Thyroid hormone increases LDL receptor expression and also enhances LPL activity. So when someone is hypothyroid, his or her LDL-c will be a bit higher than normal and oftentimes triglycerides will also be elevated due to the decreased LPL. Studies of thyroid hormone replacement for those who were previously hypothyroid show about a 10 mg/dL drop in LDL-c, and there are some studies that also show around a 20% drop in Lp(a), although this effect is variable. Additionally, hypothyroidism is a risk factor for statin-associated myopathies; essentially since your global metabolic processes are sluggish, the drug can remain in your system longer and potentially lead to increased side effects. Overall, the effects of thyroid hormone replacement on lipid levels are quite modest, and if your baseline

cholesterol metrics are stratospheric AND you're concurrently hypothyroid, you're probably not going to be living in that much safer of a Lipid Neighborhood even if your thyroid gets properly regulated.

6. **So if I'm truly hypothyroid, what do I do about it?**
    a. As clinicians, I think we all need to be comfortable with the various options for thyroid hormone replacement. Some people do wonderfully on T4 monotherapy, while others take T4 plus a separate dose of T3. Some people feel horrible on T4 alone, but thrive on desiccated pig thyroid, which is a combination product of both T4 and T3. Under normal physiologic circumstances, your body makes around 100 mcg of T4 and around 30 mcg of T3, and most of the T3 is converted from T4. Some people are "bad converters," so they might need a little more T3. And some people might convert the T4 to T3 just fine. Sometimes it takes a little trial and error to find the right approach for people, but being a "Synthroid monogamist" is a good way to have everyone hate you as a practitioner.
7. **What about "Thyroid Support" supplements?**
    a. Well, a lot of times these supplements actually have either T4, T3, or both in the "mystery proprietary blend." It's sort of like Red Yeast Rice...people think they're being "natural" and they're just taking an unregulated, highly variable dose of a prescription medication. And a lot of times these supplements have supraphysiologic doses of iodine, which can really screw things up. While it's true the body needs iodine to synthesize thyroid hormones, if you take too much iodine, one of two disastrous situations can result (and you know it's bad because both of these conditions have HYPHENS). Excess iodine

can result in either the Wolf-Chaikoff effect or the Jod-Basedow phenomenon. Remember, iodine is like the chocolate chips in the thyroid hormone cookies, and if you have way too many chocolate chips, you can either stop making cookies (Wolf-ChaikOFF... you turn OFF thyroid hormone production and become hypothyroid) or you make A LOT MORE COOKIES and become hyperthyroid (Jod-Basedow). Either way, it's a dumb idea. I had several patients develop goiters due to excessive iodine supplementation, and unless you're going for that "I swallowed an avocado and it got stuck midway down my throat look," that's probably not what you want out of your "Thyroid Support."

8. **And what about tyrosine, selenium, and biotin?**
   a. I don't think a lack of tyrosine is the reason why anyone is hypothyroid, since it's the precursor for both thyroid hormones and catecholamines and is derived from phenylalanine anyway. And while selenium does assist in the conversion of T4 to T3 (and a couple Brazil nuts do have your recommended daily dose) and it may be worth supplementing in certain instances, it's pretty much like trying to douse a forest fire with a squirt gun if your TSH is 35 and you haven't had a bowel movement for 10 days. Biotin doesn't actually affect your thyroid at all, but it can mess with your lab results, which is why it's recommended to stop biotin supplementation a few days before drawing thyroid function tests.

Well, that was fun...and now against my better judgment I'll briefly discuss "Adrenal Fatigue," although the mere thought is admittedly exhausting.

Adrenal Fatigue

I've had plenty of patients come to me having been told by a "holistic practitioner" that they had "adrenal fatigue." Well, your adrenals aren't ovaries, and most organs don't reach a certain age where they just stop working (unless you're dead). Unlike menopause, there is no Pancreo-Pause (although your pancreas certainly hates you if you're eating the Standard American Diet). There is no Brain-o-Pause (although many Junior High boys are at least making this a debatable point). So let's discuss adrenal physiology for a minute here and put to rest this myth of Adrenal Fatigue, which would be better described as "Hypothalamic-Pituitary-Adrenal Axis Dysfunction." Just saying that mouthful more than once is fatiguing, but let's press on.

The adrenal glands are like a couple of jelly donuts that sit on top of the kidneys; the cortex is the outer layer and the jelly in the middle is the adrenal medulla. Normally, your hypothalamus produces corticotropin-releasing hormone (CRH), which signals the anterior pituitary to produce adrenocorticotropic hormone (ACTH), which then signals the adrenal glands to produce cortisol from a layer of the cortex called the zona fasciculata. (The adrenal cortex also produces aldosterone and DHEA from the zona glomerulosa and reticularis, respectively, and the medulla produces catecholamines like norepinephrine and epinephrine). However, the primary player in regulating this feedback loop is cortisol.

Cortisol is similar to insulin in that a lack of cortisol is incompatible with life, but excess cortisol makes it impossible to have any semblance of metabolic health. People with autoimmune destruction of the adrenal gland, or Addison's Disease, need lifelong replacement of cortisol and aldosterone or else they die. (Interestingly, President JFK had Addison's Disease). Conversely, people with a pathologic excess of cortisol, called Cushing's, cannot "Control their insulin, control their life" even if they're doing all the right things. That's because excess cortisol is catabolic to muscle, anabolic to fat, leaves them "tired but wired," and progressively ruins their lives unless they are appropriately diagnosed and treated. The classic Cushing's phenotype is someone who resembles Dr. Robotnik from the original Sonic the Hedgehog games...comically thin extremities with truncal obesity, purple stretch marks, perpetually flushed cheeks even in the absence of embarrassing life situations, and a fatty hump that would make all the buffaloes on the Wyoming plains jealous. Additionally, these folks often have resistant hypertension and poorly controlled blood sugars until either the pituitary or adrenal tumor that is sabotaging their metabolism is addressed.

However, the diagnosis of Cushing's is rarely this straightforward. For instance, I had a patient who was a total rock star; she was literally doing ALL THE RIGHT THINGS that would normally lead to metabolic optimization. However, her lipid profile was characterized by low HDL-c and elevated fasting triglycerides. Despite working out like a fiend, she was prediabetic and hypertensive. And despite eating a monastically clean diet, she continued to steadily gain fat mass around the abdomen. And guess what? She had an adrenal adenoma, and within 6 months of its removal her physique and labs matched her lifestyle, which was amazing.

So do we need to screen every single American for Cushing's? Obviously not. But there are several situations where I would encourage clinicians to be comfortable obtaining either a late-night salivary cortisol or low-dose dexamethasone suppression test as screening tests for cortisol excess:

- The person has "chicken legs" and abdominal obesity.
- The person has poorly controlled diabetes on multiple medications.
- The person has a dyslipidemic and insulin resistant

blood profile despite TRULY pulling all the right levers when it comes to lifestyle.

And do we need to screen every single American for "Adrenal Fatigue?" Well, if it existed, then maybe. And does non-pathologic "Adrenal Dysfunction" contribute to feelings of tiredness and suboptimal quality of life? Sure. And if you have been diagnosed with "Adrenal Fatigue," the solution is to identify the stressors in your life and find a way to manage those factors. Easier said than done, but all the ashwagandha, rhodiola, and Holy Basil in the world won't help your situation unless you can find ways to navigate the stressful tyranny of life triumphantly.

2

THE DARK ARTS OF HORMONE REPLACEMENT THERAPY

"We don't talk enough about the risks of NOT considering hormone therapy...it's not just the risk of taking menopausal hormone therapy that we need to consider."
-Rachel Rubin, MD

When I was in High School, my English teacher tasked us with a "fun" assignment to write a paper about our family traditions. Given that "eating turkey on Thanksgiving" and "unwrapping presents at Christmas" struck me as unworthy topics on which to expend my mellifluous prose, I instead fabricated an outrageous narrative fraught with hilarious caricatures and unbelievable anecdotes. Pleased with my work, I volunteered to share my essay with the class. I'm pretty sure that several intercostal injuries were sustained from the peals of laughter and it's possible that the local Richter scale detected a few mirth-quakes in the aftermath of the dramatic reading.

My teacher, however, failed to share in the jocularity and gave me a zero on the paper. But right around that same time, I was applying to various colleges. Typically with these applications I would have to submit an utterly banal essay about why I wanted to go to college and what I eventually wanted to do with my career or something similarly lame. But Texas Christian University, who had not previously been on my radar but had waived my application fee, simply said, "Submit us a copy of what you consider your best work."

So, covering up the conspicuous red "Zero" at the top of my Family Traditions paper, I submitted my essay to the TCU admissions office; despite the lack of pedagogical appreciation, I still thought that this was pretty much the zenith of my literary undertakings at the time. And you know what? They offered me their full-ride scholarship worth over $85,000 if I were to matriculate and major in Broadcast Journalism. Take that, teacher who will remain unnamed!

I didn't end up accepting their offer, but admit it...it's kind of fun to fantasize about what could have been! I bet you'd at least consider tuning in if I were commentating alongside Tom Brady in the broadcast booth or pontificating with Stephen A. Smith about who's the greatest basketball player of all time...but we'll never know.

Somewhat similarly, we will never fully know the exact best way to approach the "Dark Arts" of postmenopausal hormone replacement therapy (HRT) based on the "Gold Standard" of randomized controlled trials. However, I do feel we can make reasonable speculations based on historical observations and the available information to intervene appropriately on an individualized basis.

In the RIGHT PERSON at the RIGHT TIME with the RIGHT REGIMEN I feel that HRT can have a net benefit in not only bone health, but also long-term cardiovascular and brain health.

However, in the WRONG PERSON at the WRONG TIME with the WRONG REGIMEN, post-menopausal HRT could exacerbate underlying cardiovascular disease. So let's briefly discuss some mechanisms of HRT and some trials that could help better inform our treatment decisions when it comes to this patient population.

So one of the big issues with many of the HRT trials is that they used something called Conjugated Equine Estrogen, or CEE. Savvy wordsmiths will recognize "equine" as a word that means "pertaining to horses." And CEE is literally a "mystery proprietary blend" of 10 different estrogens harvested from the urine of pregnant horses. I mean, horses ARE majestic creatures and they do pee a lot, so why not use a gravid mare's ample secretions as a way to mitigate hot flashes? You can't make this stuff up.

Clearly we have better options these days (various "bioidentical" and transdermal formulations, for instance), but these were not available at the time these studies were performed. So we have to do our best with pregnant horse pee data (I almost threw in an "oral" there as well, but that seemed like too much).

Another variable is that many of these studies involved synthetic progestin formulations rather than oral micronized progesterone. If individuals still have a uterus during HRT, some type of progesterone must be supplemented along with the estrogen in order to avoid endometrial hyperplasia. However, progestins are notorious for causing off-target effects, including weight gain, potential worsening of insulin resistance, and even elevations in LDL cholesterol. So there's another cook in the complicated kitchen.

Despite these factors, the results of the Women's Health Initiative (WHI), which utilized both CEE and medroxyprogesterone acetate, a synthetic progestin, were still arguably inconclusive in regards to cardiovascular health. The WHI was littered with individuals who would not have been good candidates for HRT at baseline (due to factors such as smoking and having gone through menopause over a decade prior to intervention), but in subanalysis of women under age 60, there was still a 40% reduction in heart attacks for that cohort. A meta-analysis of randomized controlled trials in women under 60 and HRT initiated within 10 years of menopause showed a 32% reduction in coronary disease as well as a 39% reduction in all-cause mortality.

Additionally, another trial using oral estrogen, the ELITE trial, showed that, when started early in the menopausal transition, carotid intimal medial thickness progression was stultified...but there was no apparent benefit when started later. And the Danish Osteoporosis Prevention study showed a 52% reduction in heart attacks, heart failure, and death when HRT was initiated in younger females within 7 months of being classified as postmenopausal. These individuals were followed for 16 years and there was no increase in cancers, strokes, or blood clots, either. Similarly, an Icelandic study of those who started HRT early in the menopausal transition had a >50% lower average CAC than those who never initiated treatment when followed over 15 years. Go Scandinavia!

And although we know that synthetic progestins are about as dirty as a Motley Crue concert, the jury is still out on whether oral or transdermal estrogen is the best choice; it likely depends on the individual. The KEEPS trial showed us that either transdermal or oral estrogen seem to be safe when combined with intermittent oral progesterone from a cardiovascular standpoint. The women in this study had pretty decent Home Security Systems; their HOMA-IR values were normal and they had unremarkable measures of systemic inflammation like hs-CRP and even IL-6. And the few women with some CAC in that study (although all had CAC values <50) didn't trend in the wrong direction with either oral or transdermal formulations over the

4-year follow-up period. I would've loved to see them measure Lp(a) in that study.

So what do we make of all this? Well, estrogen is an insulin sensitizer, and no one ever said, "Boy, I wish I was more insulin resistant." Estrogen plays a role in inhibiting PCSK9, and we would prefer our LDL receptor claw grabbers to remain in working order instead of being put "out of commission" by excessive PCSK9. Estrogen also inhibits something called SR-B1, which is one of the "roads" of transcytosis by which ApoB mailmen can drive their trucks into your arterial wall; estrogen basically helps the mailmen go home to the liver at the end of the day. And there are other putative roles of optimal estrogen levels in everything from bone health to brain health.

So, ultimately what do I think about HRT during the menopausal transition? In the RIGHT person (which means appropriate baseline cardiovascular risk stratification, including detailed history, CAC, lipid metrics, and everything else in our Home Security System and Lipid Neighborhood framework)...

With the RIGHT formulation (estrogen and, if progesterone is used, not employing synthetic progestins, which seem to be "cleaner" options in regards to mitigating off-target effects). Whether or not oral or transdermal estrogen is employed depends on the specific symptoms that the individual may be trying to address along with genetic factors...

At the RIGHT time (not waiting until the person has been post-menopausal for over a decade)...

You may very well achieve a net benefit in regards to not only cardiovascular health, but overall quality of life. Will we ever know for sure? Probably not, but I think that we can have a nice, individualized, nuanced approach when looking at the body of data.

Oral or Transdermal Estrogen?

Well, if it were an easy answer, then we wouldn't be calling this the "Dark Arts." But consider this:

- Oral estrogen reduces ApoB, LDL-c, and Lp(a), but can increase triglycerides and can shift LDL particles to a Pattern B of predominantly small, dense species. Transdermal estrogen doesn't affect lipids much, although it may reduce Lp(a) a smidge.
- Transdermal estrogen doesn't increase sex-hormone binding globulin (SHBG), which may be useful if low libido is an issue. Increased SHBG can bind up circulating testosterone and compromise its bioavailability, which could abrogate a beneficial effect on "drive."
- Both formulations seem reasonably effective in reducing hot flashes and preserving bone mineral density.
- Transdermal estrogen is less likely to result in venous thromboembolisms (blood clots).
- Or, if the patient is solely experiencing localized systems (like vaginal atrophy or recurrent urinary tract infections), a cream may be the most appropriate intervention.

Once again, appropriately analyzing ALL the individual factors for the patient prior to making a treatment recommendation can at least help us make somewhat enlightened decisions when it comes to the Dark Arts.

Now what about testosterone?

Well, if you're a female and you're now capable of growing a mustache that Tom Selleck would envy, your voice has gone from sultry to Darth Vader-esque, and your husband "really needs a break" from your romantic advances, you've overshot things. However, many gals could probably benefit from low doses.

And for males? Well, this becomes a similar situation to post-menopausal HRT. In the right person at the right time with the right formulation, it may lead to both cardiovascular benefits and improvements in quality of life. Conversely, it's possible that it may exacerbate underlying cardiovascular disease in the wrong person at the wrong time with the wrong system of delivery. I think the issue is even more murky than post-menopausal HRT.

So what does testosterone or testosterone replacement therapy (TRT) do for you? I don't remember where I first heard this, but testosterone "makes effort feel good." If you get on the sauce and sit around watching Netflix, you're not taking advantage of an incredible performance enhancer. Conversely, if you are on TRT, it allows you to pick up heavy things, sprint, and be even more of a Spartan at life than you otherwise could be without help. Instead of having normal physiologic fluctuations in testosterone over the course of the day, you essentially remain at whatever level you've achieved if you're dosing consistently and properly.

That said, if you are a bro and you have "low T," (and low T has been associated with increased mortality in men with heart disease) let's ask a few questions about why your T may be low:

1. Is your testosterone low and are you also incapable of smelling (a condition known as anosmia) and are you still waiting to go through puberty? Then you may have Kallmann Syndrome, a rare pituitary disorder (the likelihood of this is even more unlikely than you actually NEEDING TRT if you're pulling all the right lifestyle levers and you're under age 30).

2. Is your testosterone low and are you running 100 miles a week, starving yourself, or going through Navy Seal training?
    a. Well, maybe mix in a rest day here and there or consider breaking your fast.
3. Is your testosterone low and are you drinking a bunch of alcohol?
    a. See Chapter 2 if you think that drinking alcohol is a good choice for optimal health and performance. If you stop drinking alcohol, your testosterone will inevitably go up.
4. Is your testosterone low and are you either completely sedentary, eating a Standard American Diet (SAD), not sleeping well, and overly stressed (or some combination of all of the above)?
    a. Pick up heavy things, sprint, stop eating crap, and then your subtle sleep apnea will go away too so you'll sleep better. And when you feel better, you'll probably be less stressed. And then guess what? YOU PROBABLY WON'T HAVE LOW TESTOSTERONE ANYMORE.

As far as cardiovascular health goes, if your testosterone is sky-high and you're dosing yourself with so much sauce that you have to donate blood every week, you probably ought to throttle back. A recent trial called the TRAVERSE study suggested that TRT is not harmful in regards to cardiovascular health, but it utilized a testosterone gel and they limited the levels of testosterone achieved in the patient population...so I don't think they really answered the question given they used a garbage formulation and didn't reach real-world testosterone levels. Another trial of testosterone in those with coronary plaque showed some progression of soft plaque in certain individuals...although CAC scores remained largely unchanged. In vitro studies show that testosterone may play a role in hyper-elongating glycosaminoglycan chains in the artery wall (a bunch of big words that mean potentially worsening existing cardiovascular disease). And testosterone increases hepatic lipase, leading to a temporary reduction of HDL-c; whether or not this has any meaningful physiologic consequence is unknown. Plus, if you take a bunch of TRT and never do aerobic exercise, you are likely going to experience concentric hypertrophy of your heart muscle without proper eccentric hypertrophy to balance things out. Which can result in elevated blood pressure and other cardiac dysfunction.

So do you need TRT? Probably not. Will it help you pull the levers to be a champion in life? Possibly, but maybe you should first just try to do those things anyway. And then if you're still low, do some baseline cardiovascular risk stratification and then maybe consider it. I've prescribed TRT on many occasions and I'm not opposed to it, but I think it's often overused and employed irresponsibly.

I went through some very serious illnesses and my total testosterone plummeted as low as 70. Did I feel good? Nope. And I was even on TRT for a brief time. But I tapered off of it and now I sit around 900. How did I do this? Picked up heavy things. Sprinted. Didn't eat crap or drink alcohol. Slept. Day after day.

One of my favorite studies enrolled guys who unfortunately had to be on androgen deprivation therapy for prostate cancer (you have to drive your testosterone levels down to zero in order to sensitize the prostate to radiation). And these guys had testosterone levels of VIRTUALLY ZERO...I'd say that's "Low T." And the group that continued to resistance train experienced NO LOSS IN MUSCLE MASS despite having the lowest T ever. Did their "effort feel good?" I guarantee they felt like death...I've been there. But they manned up and decided that it's better to feel like crap and be strong than to feel like crap and be weak. Kudos to those guys, and I think that should serve as inspiration for all of us to be good stewards of our hormonal health.

3

OXYTOCIN

"You know you're in love when you can't fall asleep because reality is finally better than your dreams."
-Dr. Seuss

Oxytocin...the LOVE HORMONE. And since we LOVE our Home Security System and our Lipid Neighborhood, I think it's worth paying homage to this seldom-studied posterior pituitary hormone. There are a few interesting studies of oxytocin showing both some beneficial effects on insulin sensitivity and lowering of LDL cholesterol. One really intriguing short study using an intranasal oxytocin formulation in older adults improved lean muscle mass and lowered LDL-c 19%. Gotta love that!

But one reason I bring up oxytocin is that I had a patient who came to me complaining of hot flashes...and the menopausal train had left the station about 25 years prior to me seeing her. Intervening with any sort of HRT wasn't an option, and I wasn't particularly convinced that her new complaint was even related to the Dark Arts hormones. So I figured I would placate her by running some really esoteric labs to rule out serotonin-producing carcinoid tumors and other stuff I knew she didn't have. I was confident that a deluge of sesquipedalian medical jargon would douse any last vestiges of her hot flashes, but after I explained all the tests I ran and the scary things she didn't have, she was unimpressed. "So what are you gonna do for me?" she asked curtly. Honestly at a loss for any legitimate suggestion beyond trial-and-error off-label antidepressant use (which would have sent her into an apoplectic rage), I called up my buddy at the local pharmacy and had him compound some sublingual oxytocin lozenges...I figured it wouldn't hurt, and at least I was doing SOMETHING. And it CHANGED HER LIFE...and now she goes around telling all her friends, family, and random strangers that they should get some oxytocin lozenges. Genius stuff, right?!

But the ACTUAL reason I mention oxytocin in a book about lipids? It gives me an excuse to share a legitimate Love Story with you all...sometimes real life is even better than fairytales!

How I Met My Wife

Life is a constellation of beautiful stories, and one story that I never get tired of purveying is the tale of how my wife and I met. Similar to many fairytales and romance novels, we first saw each other in front of a U-Haul; we had both been recruited to help a mutual friend move across town. I was nattily clad in a baseball tournament shirt from when I was 11 years old (I'm still waiting for that magical growth spurt), and she was all dolled up in a purple tie-dye shirt brandishing a utility knife. Despite our stunning wardrobes, it was actually her confidence that immediately stood out to me; she was completely comfortable in her own skin (and tie-dye shirt), and this was intriguing to me given the annoying engulfment of insecurity that often renders physically attractive people intolerably insipid. I later found out that she was also packing a Taser and pepper spray, and perhaps these elements contributed to her self-assuredness.

But anyway, delightful dialogue ensued and persisted as we trafficked boxes and furniture in and out of the U-Haul. And at the end of the night, I said to the group, "Guys, this has really been fun...I'd like to get all your phone numbers so we can all hang out again!" Now, did I really care about scoring Carl's number or feel any rush of excitement as I pretended to enter Jamie's digits into my first-generation flip phone? Clearly not, but I thought it was a pretty slick and non-confrontational way to secure the vivacious olive-skinned girl's contact information...after all, I still needed to be wary of her Taser and pepper spray.

I knew on Day 6 I was going to marry her. During that time I was finishing up my first Doctorate, so I was driving back and forth from Boise to Pocatello multiple times per week, because although I was physically going to school in Eastern Idaho, my heart was 3 and a half hours west. And on one of those drives, waves of inspiration flooded my lovestruck brain, and the result of this deluge was some lyrics to a song...not a rap, but a song asking this girl to marry me. So I pulled over at Exit 208 outside of a town called Burley, sprinted into a gas station, grabbed a napkin and a pen, and furiously jotted down the passionate poetry.

And, as the story unfolds, those lyrics must have been pretty good. Because right before I proposed to her, I decided, after careful consideration, that it probably would be best to NOT wear the baseball shirt from when I was 11 years old when I asked her the most important question of my life. And given that my hair, which could euphemistically be described as "lush and voluminous" would more accurately be described as "undomesticated and utterly incapable of being tamed," I felt it would be appropriate to get a haircut as well.

And I usually give the barber a picture of Zac Efron or Rob Lowe and say, "Do that," and typically it sort of works out ok and then I can pomade my way to aesthetic acceptability. However, on this occasion, the barber at Not-So-Great Clips practically sheared me; I have never received anything that close to a buzz cut in my life. And this is a massive problem; I have a comically small and weirdly-shaped head; this is why I need ample plumage to conceal this horrifying secret.

So there I was, 3 days before the biggest moment of my life, and my lopsided light-bulb of a head had nowhere to hide; I had to hope that "my nice personality" and ability to play guitar would overshadow the abomination above my eyebrows. So I rented a U-Haul, decorated it in a florally festive manner, left my guitar in there, parked the truck at some friends' house, picked up some of the Youth Group kids from church to further set up the ruse that we were helping some people move...and when I opened up the door to the U-Haul, I got down and played that song. And I guess it worked! But boy, that haircut was truly a test of her unconditional love; those pictures of me from that day simultaneously evoke pity and nausea.

If you get married, don't settle for anything less than marrying your best friend, even if they've just gotten a cringeworthy haircut. And she is, without a doubt, my best friend, and I thank God every day that He brought us together; I couldn't live without her.

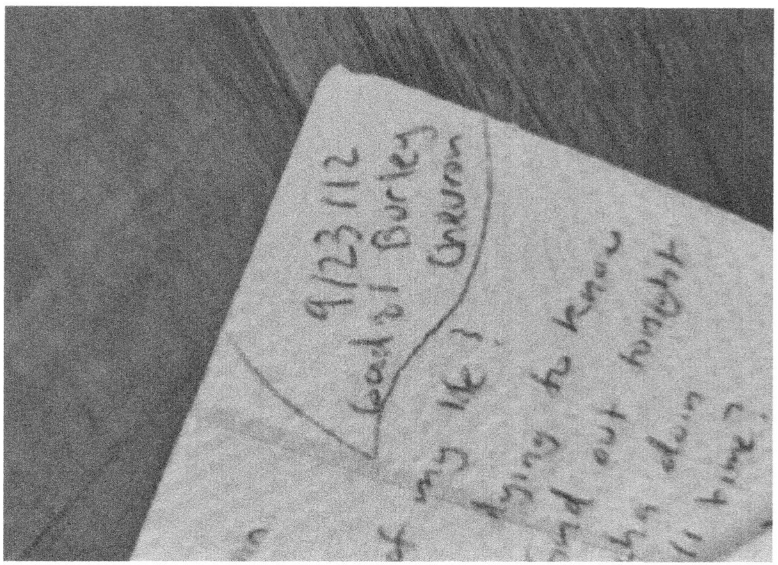

That napkin has been forever immortalized! Oh you wanted to see the lyrics? That's not for you...my heart (and any napkins with pieces of my heart) only belong to her.

4

PROLACTIN, GROWTH HORMONE, AND PARATHYROID HORMONE

"Got milk?"
-Ridiculous slogan from the 1990s accompanied by various celebrities featuring comically inappropriate white mustaches

Prolactin

Prolactin is a fascinating hormone. If you possess the requisite anatomical machinery for milk production and are currently breastfeeding, then you'll have "physiologic" hyperprolactinemia. Conversely, if you've acquired the nickname, "The Milkman" and have resorted to wearing highly-absorbent sweatshirts in public settings, you probably have already gone to your doctor.

However, more subtle elevations in prolactin (which are generally the case with a pituitary microadenoma) can lead to perturbations in your lipid panel; hyperprolactinemia often causes elevated LDL-c, high triglycerides, and low HDL-c. Additionally, it can be accompanied by low testosterone. I had several young male patients with previously unexplained low testosterone and a lipid panel that just didn't match their overall lifestyle habits who had prolactin-secreting pituitary tumors, so keep hyperprolactinemia in mind for those sorts of situations. And oftentimes treating the patient with a dopamine-receptor agonist like cabergoline will normalize both the low testosterone and the lipid anomalies. There is some REALLY complicated interplay between dopamine and prolactin, both in the brain and in peripheral fat cells, that likely contributes to the metabolic and lipid disturbances seen in hyperprolactinemia. This is why dopamine BLOCKERS like Olanzapine and Clozapine (used in conditions such as schizophrenia) often result in secondary hyperprolactinemia and accompanying lipid disturbances as well.

Growth Hormone

Deficiencies in growth hormone can result in a dysmetabolic Lipid Panel of low HDL-c and high triglycerides, while growth hormone excess can lead to a marked increase in Lp(a). Additionally, treatment with Growth Hormone can significantly increase levels of Lp(a). So if you're an athlete who "knows people" as you attempt a superhuman recovery from your torn meniscus, it's probably not a great idea to remain on the HGH sauce long-term, if at all. Doing something of questionable legality that increases the Felons of the Lipid Neighborhood doesn't strike me as the best idea from a cardiovascular risk standpoint.

Parathyroid Hormone

Parathyroid hormone (PTH) is the master regulator of calcium homeostasis, and very commonly folks will have secondary hyperparathyroidism due to chronic kidney disease and/or vitamin D deficiency. These folks will have elevated PTH but normal calcium levels. But in PRIMARY hyperparathyroidism both PTH and calcium will be concurrently elevated. Although primary hyperparathyroidism can result in the classic "kidney stones, groans (from GI distress) and psychiatric moans" symptoms, it's important to also recognize that chronic elevations in PTH can also elevate blood pressure. This is likely due to calcium's central role in optimizing muscular contraction, including cardiac and smooth muscle contraction, along with some more complex mechanisms involving interplay between calcium homeostasis and aldosterone.

But the REAL reason I bring up PTH is because of the "Athlete's Paradox" in which we observe elevated coronary plaques in athletes participating in long-term, high-intensity extreme endurance exercise (think Tour de France, marathon running, and Ironman Triathlons). There are multiple studies showing both elevated CAC and elevated mixed plaques in those with the highest levels of lifelong high-intensity endurance exercise volume when compared to age and risk-factor matched controls. However, there are many limitations to these studies and much heterogeneity; in the same study showing that male athletes were 22% more likely to have coronary plaque than their less-extreme male counterparts, there was no difference among female athletes versus the control group. And we still don't really have any data on these groups when it comes to actually having clinical events like heart attacks and strokes...there is much to learn.

So why do some of these Mitochondrial Mavens have advanced atherosclerosis? Well, I think it ultimately comes down to an inability to make a beneficial adaptation to a chronically imposed stressor. At some point, probably due to many other individual genetic factors, we can all reach our tipping point when it comes to resilience. However, one plausible hormonal mechanism for this phenomenon is elevated levels of PTH; PTH rises dramatically in response to intense exercise, and if these elite athletes are "burning the candle too hot" for too long without adequate recovery in their training regimens, it's possible that this could accelerate vascular calcification.

So should you use this an excuse to be sedentary? I think you would have stopped reading this book long before this section if you were trying to justify being a slug. But it appears that just like everything else, there can, even with exercise, be too much of a good thing. The same intrinsic drive that can make you a superstar can, perhaps, also be your downfall...believe me, I've been there myself when it comes to exercise addiction and over-training. It almost cost me my life. But kept in balance, the gift of movement is perhaps the greatest intervention that any of us can utilize to optimize cardiovascular health and virtually every facet of our well-being.

PART IV

THE DEEP END OF THE COMMUNITY POOL

1

CONDITIONS OF LOW HDL CHOLESTEROL

"Get low, get low, get low, get low"
-Lil' Jon and the East Side Boyz,
allegedly in reference to ApoA-1 Milano

If you're studying for your Lipid Boards, then get ready for a plunge into some rare pathologies!

Tangier Disease

When I first started learning about Tangier Disease, I was brimming with excitement; I was almost certain that the stored knowledge of capitals and major cities of every African country that I had memorized in 2nd grade was finally going to come in handy (since I had long been aware that, along with Rabat and Casablanca, Tangier was one of Morocco's major metropolitan areas). And to my dismay, I found out that Tangier is actually a weird island in Chesapeake Bay best known for soft-shell crabs. Life is full of crushing disappointments.

Tangier Disease is a genetic defect in the ABCA1 gene. And without ABCA1, HDL particles can't acquire cholesterol. So with Tangier Disease, these people will have nearly undetectable HDL-c levels, typically less than 5 mg/dL (although they will have some ApoA-1). Additionally, since ABCA1 plays a pivotal role in transporting cholesterol out of macrophages into HDL particles, the cholesterol instead accumulates in various macrophage-rich tissues such as the spleen and liver; this results in hepatosplenomegaly. However, the most well-known feature of Tangier Disease is ORANGE TONSILS, since the tonsils are also a lymphoid tissue. Just remember T for Tonsils and you'll be golden (or orange).

People with Tangier Disease often are plagued with neurological disorders, but they don't always get cardiovascular disease. I've only known one person with this disease, and that person was astonishingly underwhelmed when I started discussing soft-shell crabs and cities in Morocco. People are strange sometimes.

So for Tangier Disease, which is a very popular topic on board exams:

- Defect in ABCA1
- HDL-c <5, detectable ApoA-1
- ORANGE TONSILS, hepatosplenomegaly, peripheral neuropathy

Familial Hypoalphalipoproteinemia

This is another condition of low HDL-c that, in contrast to Tangier Disease, is characterized by undetectable ApoA-1. These folks also are riddled with premature coronary disease and may also have tendinous xanthomas. The defect here is a mutation in the *APOA1* gene on Chromosome 11. Big-time bummer.

Familial LCAT Deficiency and Fish-Eye Disease

As you will recall, one of the other key components in HDL maturation (along with ApoA-1 and ABCA1) is LCAT; this enzyme esterifies the cholesterol that is effluxed into the HDL particle. However, without the capacity to properly esterify the acquired cholesterol in Familial LCAT Deficiency, the HDL particle is targeted for degradation by the kidney, leading to HDL-c levels less than 10. Also, something called Lipoprotein X accumulates, which itself is nephrotoxic (more on Lipoprotein X in the Bile Acid section...just remember X for toXic for now). And the kidney becomes OVERWHELMED as it attempts to catabolize all the ApoA-1 while also dealing with the Lipoprotein X. Unfortunately, this condition leads to progressive kidney disease that will eventually necessitate transplant. Additionally, these individuals have premature coronary disease, hemolytic anemia, and corneal opacities (with such low HDL-c they can't "c" straight).

A less severe version of Familial LCAT Deficiency is called "Fish Eye Disease." These people are able to avoid the severe kidney disease and other horribly debilitating symptoms of LCAT Deficiency, but their eyes just resemble a fish. Glub glub. So for Familial LCAT Deficiency and Fish Eye Disease:

- Genetic loss of function in LCAT
- HDL-c levels <10
- Progressive kidney disease, premature ASCVD, hemolytic anemias, corneal opacities
- Fish Eye Disease: Less severe, just weird fish eyes, may need corneal transplant

ApoA-1 Milano

There are certain people of Italian descent with incredibly low HDL-c levels who apparently have a "superpowered" HDL dubbed ApoA-1 Milano. These folks are seemingly immune to cardiovascular disease despite these low HDL-c levels and don't appear to have other issues. A similar variant resulting in low but seemingly highly functional HDL-c called ApoA-1 Paris has also been identified (and this is not the Paris in Idaho...it's actually what you think). HDL is crazy!

Disappearing HDL Syndrome

Rarely there can be an interaction between medications that results in very low HDL-c levels. One of these causes of "Disappearing HDL Syndrome" can occur when someone is on both a thiazolidinedione (TZD) and a fibrate simultaneously. Why does this happen? I could make something up that would sound plausible regarding interplay between various nuclear transcription factors, but we don't really know. This phenomenon was also recently observed in a patient on both bempedoic acid and a fibrate. So there's something funky about those fibrates!

2

CONDITIONS OF LOW LDL CHOLESTEROL

"I've got friends in low places"
-Garth Brooks, purportedly in reference to several acquaintances with hypobetalipoproteinemia

As stated previously, every nucleated cell in your body synthesizes its own cholesterol. And if your plasma cholesterol is low, it matters WHY it's low. If you have sepsis and/or are actively dying, then that's not so good. If your complexion resembles a lemon and you have end-stage liver disease, your LDL-c will be low for less-than-ideal reasons. And if you have abetalipoproteinemia, as we will discuss, then that's also problematic. But if you have a genetic loss-of-function in PCSK9 or ANGPTL3, then you're probably fine and have a lower risk of coronary disease. Context always matters!

Abetalipoproteinemia (also known as Bassen-Kornzweig Syndrome if you're into hyphens and impressing people with large Austrian words)

Basically, these individuals are unable to equip the ApoB mailmen with triglyceride cargo due to a genetic defect in microsomal triglyceride transfer protein (MTTP), so delivery of triglycerides, fat soluble vitamins, and phospholipids is SEVERELY IMPAIRED. Their plasma ApoB is undetectable. Consequently, these individuals have horrible malabsorptive diarrhea, profound deficiency in vitamins A, D, E, and K, terrible neurologic issues such as spinocerebellar ataxia, and a nasty eye condition called retinitis pigmentosa. If these kiddos don't get some immediate help, they're not going to survive for very long. A similar condition called Chylomicron Retention Disease due to a defect in SAR1B GTPase results in the same phenotype.

Hypobetalipoproteinemia

Conversely, those with hypobetalipoproteinemia, often due to a truncated ApoB-100, have lifelong low levels of ApoB (usually <40 mg/dL), but are generally asymptomatic. Occasionally they will have a slight deficiency in some fat-soluble vitamins, and they are predisposed to fatty liver due to triglyceride "packages" accumulating in the liver. Their "postprandial chylomicron mailmen" do their jobs normally, but the "VLDL/IDL/LDL mailmen who work around the clock" don't really deliver the mail very well. These people rarely get atherosclerotic vascular disease since they live in a very safe Lipid Neighborhood...but there are case reports of people with hypobetalipoproteinemia having coronary disease. And guess what? THEY HAD DIABETES. So even in an idyllic pastoral setting with very few Lipid Criminals, crimes can still be committed if your Home Security System has made your arterial abode resemble an abandoned shack.

Low LDL Cholesterol and All-Cause Mortality

But Josh, haven't you seen the studies that show an INCREASED risk of mortality with low LDL cholesterol and/or ApoB? Yep! And this is another situation in which it matters WHY your LDL-c or ApoB is low. On several occasions, I obtained a Lipid Panel on my patients and their ApoB and LDL-c was DRAMATICALLY reduced from its baseline...and on both occasions, the patients had life-threatening illnesses. And in conditions of severe malnutrition, sepsis, or any situation in which you're on Death's Doorstep, cholesterol metrics will be low. So this is yet another case in which one biomarker in isolation doesn't give you the full picture.

In these instances, a composite metric called the Metabolic Vulnerability Index, or MVX, could perhaps better inform us of the individual's risk for mortality. MVX includes 4 measures of nutritional status: isoleucine, leucine, and valine, which are well-known among Gym Bros as the branched-chain amino acids, and a separate measurement of citrate. MVX also includes the inflammatory marker GlycA plus a quantification of small HDL particles. Those with high baseline MVX scores and increased MVX scores over time tended to have increased risk of all-cause mortality in several studies, and this metric may help capture risk of death that markers such as ApoB may not fully convey.

So, as always, context matters. If your LDL-c is low because you're ensuring the ApoB mailmen are going home at the end of the day (like those with loss-of-function PCSK9), that's a much different situation than a depleted and overwhelmed workforce in an economy that is rapidly crashing (impending death). If there aren't many mailmen on the roads at any given time, it could be due to simple efficiency; they delivered their packages and went home early. Alternatively, the workforce could have been wiped out in a septic tsunami or victimized by a cataclysmic cancer; you simply don't know without appreciating the broader context.

3

BILE ACIDS BROUGHT TO YOU BY THE LETTER 'X'!

"To think too much is a disease"
-Fyodor Dostoevsky, who wisely avoided excessive rumination about the pathophysiology of biliary disorders

A large proportion of cholesterol is utilized in bile acid synthesis, and although bile acids serve as potent signaling molecules in addition to their critical role in digestion, we will focus on a few key points related to regulation of bile production. And to keep it (sort of) simple, we will try to use the letter X as much as possible!

- **Farnesoid X Receptor,** or **FXR**, is the key bile acid sensor in the body. When levels of bile acids are high, FXR downregulates genes related to bile acid synthesis such as CYP7A1 and CYP8B1.
- The committed enzymatic step in the classical pathway of bile acid synthesis, encoded by CYP7A1, is **7-alpha hydroxylase.**
- There is an alternative pathway of bile acid synthesis that is catalyzed by the mitochondrial enzyme **27-**

hydroxylase (encoded by CYP27A1), and a defect in 27-hydroxylase leads to the genetic disorder **cerebrotendinous xanthomatosis,** or **CTX**, which is a pediatric disorder that you DON'T WANT TO MISS.

- CTX is characterized by the following:
  - Diarrhea (like the patient is taking laxatives, although they're really not)
  - Tendinous xanthomas often at extensor tendons
  - Catarax (I promise I'm good at spelling, but CTX should be high on the differential diagnosis list for any kiddo who has cataracts coupled with gastrointestinal symptoms)
  - Neurological symptoms, including ataxia
- The reason why CTX occurs is that without 27-hydroxylase, cholesterol is converted to cholestanol and bile alcohols rather than bile acids. Cholestanol, which is quite toxic, then accumulates in plasma and tissues, including the brain. Thus, plasma levels of cholesterol in those with CTX will usually be normal, but plasma cholestanol and urinary bile alcohols will be SKY-HIGH.
- Early identification is key, as initiating treatment with chenodeoxycholic acid can be life-saving and prevent neurologic deterioration.

In conditions involving the hepatobiliary tree (such as gall stones, primary biliary cholangitis, and others) you may see ABSOLUTELY STRATOSPHERIC blood cholesterol levels due to the accumulation of **Lipoprotein X**. The person's blood levels will look like they have homozygous FH, but if you check an ApoB, it will be pretty low because Lipoprotein X doesn't contain ApoB. I've seen this a few times in people with biliary obstruction. (There's also a Lipoprotein Z that can manifest in hepatobiliary issues, but Lp(Z) has an ApoB...lipids are CRAZY)!

RACQUET SPORTS, HUMILITY, AND LONGEVITY

It's important to make time for leisure activities, so let's take a quick detour to the Neighborhood Racquetball Court before we resume our time in the Deep End of the Community Pool...

I was 19 years old and at the pinnacle of my mitochondrial powers. I'm pretty sure my GPA was higher than my body fat percentage, and there wasn't a shred of doubt in my mind that I could dominate any athletic event as long as it didn't involve skates. I needed a large dose of humility, and, quite surprisingly, it was Professor Reg Cavendry who administered that bolus of ego-crushing elixir.

I had started playing racquetball, and because I was annihilating all the other student-athletes, I was under the delusion I was actually good. And unbeknownst to me, Reg had been observing these amateurish competitions with keen interest and called me up to his desk after Biomechanics class one day. "I notice you've been playing racquetball," Reg said, "And I think you and I should play." Internally, I scoffed, but looking for any excuse to skip British Poetry class, I accepted his invitation. If the basketball players and track guys couldn't score on me, then Reg didn't have a prayer. Or so I thought.

If a roughly 5-foot tall potato dumpling donned a headband and some tube socks, that would be a fairly reasonable depiction of Reg's physique. I'm not a tall guy, and I towered over him as we strolled towards Racquetball Court #2.

Over the next hour, I think I may have scored twice. I scurried around the court diving in a fruitlessly frenzied manner as Reg sprayed the court with relentless corner kill shots while barely taking a step. My ego drowned that day in a puddle of sweat, and I'm pretty sure Reg's headband was bone-dry.

But along with those hearty helpings of humility, Reg inspired in me a love of racquet sports; I feel there is an unquantifiably healthful social element that accompanies the multifaceted physical benefits of this wonderful exercise modality. And in the Copenhagen City Heart Study, the sports associated with the greatest increase in life expectancy were, in fact, racquet sports. So grab some friends and bring a tennis racquet, a pickleball, a badminton set, or all of the above; you'll probably gain some humility and add some life to your years in the process!

4

SEVERE HYPERTRIGLYCERIDEMIA, LIPOPROTEIN LIPASE, AND CHYLOMICRONEMIA

"Hey Samantha...did you draw the patient's blood or just pour some coconut milk into a test tube?"

-What I said to my phlebotomist after I saw my first patient with chylomicronemia who ended up having triglycerides >4,000 mg/dL

One of the more common patient cases that physicians and other health care professionals approach me with is the situation of extremely elevated triglycerides. We'll say that the patient has triglycerides at least >500 and often well over 1,000 mg/dL. And these situations are due to some dysfunction in the LIPOPROTEIN LIPASE (LPL) enzyme. This enzyme is produced by both adipocytes and myocytes and is critical for either storing the triglycerides delivered from ApoB-containing lipoproteins in the fat cell or taking them up in the muscle cell for subsequent utilization. Although in very rare cases the individual may have a biallelic variant resulting in virtually complete LPL deficiency, oftentimes the patient will have a combination of genetic mutations in the following alleles:

- Lipase Maturation Factor 1 (LMF1)
- Glycosylphostatidylinositol-anchored high-density lipoprotein binding protein 1 (GPIHBP1)
    - You know when the abbreviated nomenclature (GPIHBP1) is obnoxious, the full term should probably never be uttered in public.
- Apolipoprotein C2 (APOC2)
- Apolipoprotein A5 (APOA5)

All of the above characters are important in LPL function, and oftentimes people who are heterozygous for these alleles have zero issues. However, in conditions such as insulin resistance or in the presence of excessive alcohol use or certain medications, these genetic variations can lead to profound hypertriglyceridemia and possibly even pancreatitis.

So to better understand the roles that each of these proteins play in LPL activity, we are going to envision LPL as a college instructor...we'll call him "Professor LPL."

In order for Professor LPL to enroll his "triglyceride students," he must first obtain the necessary didactic training himself, which would be analogous to LMF1. Without this critical "maturation factor" LPL will be inadequately prepared to take up triglycerides. Similarly, Professor LPL must be appropriately "anchored" in foundational scientific rigor, and GPIHBP1 functions as an anchor for LPL at the capillary endothelium where the triglyceride transaction takes place. Without this stability, adequate lipolysis cannot occur.

ApoC2 can be donated from HDL to chylomicrons, VLDL, and IDL and functions as a cofactor for LPL activity; this apolipoprotein can be seen as a guidance counselor that helps the triglycerides enroll in the adipocyte or myocyte. ApoA5 indirectly assists LPL as well by inhibiting the ANGPTL3/8 complex (which we will discuss in the next section). Essentially, ApoA5 provides scholarships and grants for the triglycerides so that they can have an opportunity to participate in Professor LPL's courses.

Additionally, Professor LPL has a little-known, non-hydrolytic role in enhancing clearance of triglyceride-rich lipoproteins (largely chylomicrons and VLDL) via the hepatic LDL receptor family. I reckon this is like when the professor writes letters of recommendation for students to help get them where they need to be on the next phase of their life journey. These non-canonical functions often fly under the proverbial radar, but are certainly important in optimizing the metabolic milieu.

However, if one or several of the factors involving LPL activity are dysfunctional, the triglyceride students may get into trouble; if they're not going to class, they just might form a "pancreatitis protest" and leave your physiologic campus in utter disarray. And you don't want that!

To recap:

- The canonical role of LPL is to incorporate triglycerides delivered from ApoB-48 and ApoB-100 lipoproteins into adipocytes and myocytes.
- LPL also has a non-hydrolytic "chaperone" role in enhancing clearance of triglyceride-rich lipoproteins in the liver.
- If various genetic factors involved in optimal LPL function are aberrant, often in the context of a "second hit" of suboptimal lifestyle factors, this can result in profoundly elevated triglycerides and risk of pancreatitis.

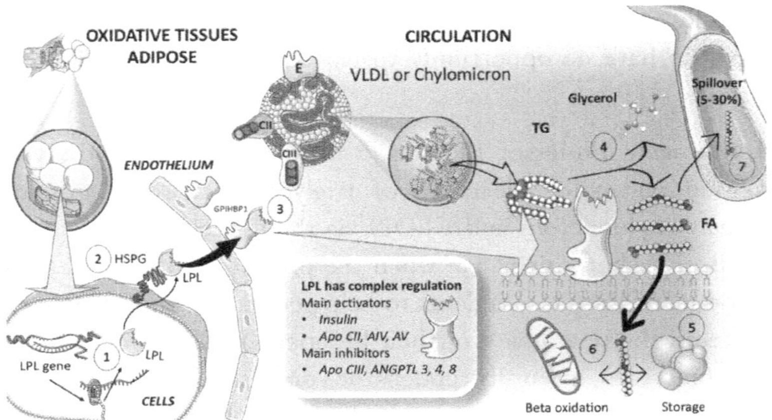

Figure 13: The Players in LPL Activity. As you can see, this is pretty convoluted, which is why Professor LPL can hopefully help you better make sense of all these regulators! Source: Gugliucci A. (2023). Sugar and dyslipidemia: A double-hit, perfect storm. *Journal of Clinical Medicine*, *12*(17), 5660. https://doi.org/10.3390/jcm12175660

Clinical Considerations

The picture used to be rather bleak for those with complete LPL deficiency or a biallelic variant resulting in virtually non-existent LPL function. This is one of the situations in which draconian fat restriction (10-15% of caloric intake) is necessary to avoid pancreatitis. Working with a dietitian to supplement with Medium Chain Triglycerides (MCTs) and other essential fatty acids while tiptoeing around the defective chylomicron transport system continues to be of paramount importance. In the past, these folks would sometimes take orlistat to inhibit fat absorption if they just couldn't resist having dessert, trading the embarrassment of fecal incontinence over hospitalization. But nowadays, we have a new drug called Olezarsen available for those with Familial Chylomicronemia Syndrome. Olezarsen is an ApoC3 inhibitor, and if you recall, ApoC3 itself is the "Great Inhibitor" of lipoprotein lipase. So by inhibiting the inhibitor, some degree of LPL function is restored.

For those who have high triglycerides without true LPL loss-of-function, oftentimes a combination of lifestyle changes and perhaps even an incretin-based therapy can effectively normalize triglycerides. I had patients with triglycerides north of 4,000 mg/dL get down to levels <150 with alcohol and fructose cessation along with a GLP-1RA to catalyze the shift to a more sustainable dietary pattern. And we didn't even have to flail around with fibrates or fish oil! Rectifying insulin resistance, stopping medications that can elevate triglycerides (such as thiazides and non-selective beta blockers), and improving lifestyle choices can make all the difference in those with Multifactorial Chylomicronemia.

BONUS COVERAGE: The ApoE Isoforms and Type III Dysbetalipoproteinemia

Recall that lipoproteins carrying ApoE have Easy and Enhanced access to the liver. Most ApoB-100 lipoproteins that have ApoE are triglyceride-rich VLDL and IDL; this is why their plasma residence time is so short compared to LDL, which lack ApoE. Interestingly, ApoE4 is actually the preferred access card to the liver...but people with ApoE4 tend to have higher levels of LDL-c. How is this possible?

Well, since VLDL and IDL particles possess FAR MORE CHOLESTEROL PER PARTICLE than LDL, the liver in ApoE4 carriers quickly satisfies its intracellular cholesterol quota and subsequently downregulates LDL receptor expression. The converse is true for ApoE2 carriers; E2 is like a poorly forged fake ID that isn't fooling anyone, so LDL receptor expression increases given that the cholesterol-rich VLDL and IDL particles with ApoE2 tend to NOT be cleared as readily. Ergo, ApoE2 carriers generally have lower LDL-c EXCEPT in rare cases of something called Type III Dysbetalipoproteinemia, or Remnant Hyperlipoproteinemia. Usually these folks are homozygotes for ApoE2, and in the presence of a "Second Hit" of insulin resistance, alcohol use, medications that impair LPL activity, or a combination of similar factors, a disastrous accumulation of triglyceride-rich remnants can result in palmar xanthomas and accelerated atherosclerosis.

This is one of the rare cases in which the majority of atherogenic lipoproteins are actually not LDL particles. Consequently, although the total cholesterol and triglycerides will be quite high in these individuals, the ApoB and directly measured LDL-c will be comparably low.

5

THE ANGPTL FAMILY

"I'm the kind of crazy you weren't warned about because no one knew this level existed"
-Usually a random girl on Instagram, but originally meant for this topic

Remember when you were a kid and you'd ask your parents some sort of question about biology or science? And your Dad would respond with a brief and either completely inaccurate or comically incomplete answer to your query...but since Dad was always right and you were probably already distracted by something else you just went along with it?

Well, the next topic on the docket is kind of similar. If you've even heard of the angiopoietin-like protein family, specifically ANGPTL3, ANGPTL4, and ANGPTL8, you've probably been told that they all inhibit lipoprotein lipase. Which is sort of true...but barely scratches the surface of their true functions. So saddle up for a discussion on the role of the ANGPTL family in FUEL PARTITIONING.

Guided by the axiom "Control your insulin, control your life," we first must recognize that insulin is the primary regulator of

ANGPTL3, ANGPTL4, and ANGPTL8. And we also must recognize that, under normal physiologic circumstances, we are meant to be cycling between fasting and fed states. When insulin is low, we ought to be in BURNING mode, partitioning fat, our savings account, toward oxidative tissues (muscles) for utilization. Conversely, when insulin is HIGH after eating, insulin directs the ingested fatty acids toward storage in fat cells to save for later. Given that LPL is the enzyme of interest in uptake of fatty acids in both adipocytes and myocytes, this provides the basis for the differing functions of ANGPTL3, ANGPTL4, and ANGPTL8 in different tissues at varying levels of insulin.

So before we talk about each individual ANGPTL member, here are a few concepts that will come in handy to reference, because this is a very complicated topic. But, if I can help your head stop spinning, this will likely result in a proverbial power plant of cognitive enlightenment once the circuitry is appropriately connected.

- ANGPTL3 and ANGPTL4 inhibit LPL.
- ANGPTL3 and ANGPTL4 form complexes with ANGPTL8. So, we can have an ANGPTL3/8 complex or an ANGPTL4/8 complex. ANGPTL8 doesn't do anything on its own, but it either amplifies the effect of ANGPTL3 or abrogates the effect of ANGPTL4 on LPL inhibition.
- ANGPTL3, ANGPTL4, and ANGPTL8 are all regulated by insulin levels.

ANGPTL3 is produced by the liver and inhibits LPL in oxidative tissues (muscle). Essentially, it partitions fatty acids toward fat cells and, when it forms a complex with ANGPTL8, further inhibits LPL in muscle. Insulin increases both ANGPTL3 and

ANGPTL8, partitioning fat toward storage in adipocytes postprandially.

ANGPTL4 is produced by adipocytes and inhibits LPL in fat cells. Consequently, ANGPTL4 is elevated during fasting, as when insulin is appropriately low, we ought to be partitioning our fatty acids toward utilization in muscle rather than storing them in fat cells. Insulin decreases ANGPTL4 and we also know that insulin increases ANGPTL8. When an ANGPTL4/8 complex is formed, it "inhibits the inhibition" of ANGPTL4 of LPL in fat cells, thus leading to increased LPL activity in the fat cell and a shift toward storage mode postprandially.

ANGPTL8 is expressed in both the liver and fat cells. It is increased by insulin levels, as stated, and is incapable of inhibiting LPL on its own.

So to recap:

- When insulin is HIGH, ANGPTL3/8 inhibits LPL in muscle and partitions fatty acids toward storage in the fat cell.
- When insulin is HIGH, ANGPTL4/8 stops inhibiting LPL in the fat cell and partitions fatty acids toward storage in the fat cell.
- When insulin is LOW, ANGPTL4 does not complex to ANGPTL8 and inhibits LPL in the fat cell, guiding fatty acids toward utilization in muscle cells.

What we just discussed was NORMAL physiologic circumstances. Under conditions of insulin resistance, we know that everything goes wrong, and there are numerous associations between chronically elevated levels of ANGPTL proteins and various disease states from obesity to diabetic retinopathy. But what's crazy is that these proteins involved in fuel partitioning actually are connected to our FIBRINOLYTIC SYSTEM (aka not throwing blood clots). Check this out!

- When an ANGPTL4/8 complex is formed, this complex binds plasminogen activator (tPA) and plasminogen to generate PLASMIN, our bodies' "clot buster."
    - Recall, ANGPTL4/8 complexes form under normal conditions of REFEEDING.
- Plasmin then degrades both ANGPTL3/8 and ANGPTL4/8 complexes, liberating LPL and restoring GLOBAL LPL ACTIVITY.
    - However, if ANGPTL4/8 complexes DO NOT FORM under conditions of refeeding, as in insulin resistance, or if the formed complex is dysfunctional, this can lead to a PROTHROMBOTIC STATE, since functional plasmin is not generated.
        - And we know that diabesity is associated with greater tendency to form blood clots of all kinds.

I bet you didn't have THAT on your Bingo card! I don't think it's particularly earth shattering to suggest that our bodies are meant to transition between fed and fasted states, but the link between EATING and CLOTTING is a twist that would possibly even surprise M. Night Shyamalan. As my Aunt Lois always says (usually in reference to a dubious link between something she ate and a sore joint): "It's ALL CONNECTED!"

6

THE INTRACELLULAR CHOLESTEROL RELAY

One of my favorite events to watch at the Summer Olympics is the 4x100 meter relay. Four of the fastest people from each country put on an otherworldly display of speed, but must also seamlessly pass the baton to one another within the transition zone in order to appropriately navigate the oval. And because of the precision required to transfer that 1.76-ounce tube (and I know a thing or two about tubes...see Appendix T), sometimes the team with the fastest individual performers fails to ascend the podium. Similarly, during the intracellular cholesterol relay, if any of the individual performers fails to "pass the cholesterol baton," things can go south in a hurry.

So we know that the LDL receptor claw grabber pulls in the LDL particle, initially forming an LDL-LDLr complex. And unless the PCSK9 hammer puts the claw grabber out of order, the LDL particle and the LDLr dissociate in the EARLY ENDOSOME, and after this dissociation the LDLr migrates back out to the cell surface to continue pulling in LDL particles. This dissociation can only occur at optimal cellular pH; this would be the starting point for "ideal racing conditions."

Once the LDL particle dissociates from the LDLr, it migrates to the LYSOSOME, which is the cellular garbage disposal, and then an enzyme called LYSOSOMAL ACID LIPASE degrades the contents of the molecule and we are left with some FREE CHOLESTEROL. Free cholesterol is the baton, and free cholesterol is the critical regulator of the genes that regulate cholesterol production, uptake, and efflux.

Coming out of the lysosomal starting blocks with the free cholesterol baton is our leadoff man, Niemann-Pick C2 (NPC2). This is different than NPC1L1, which is the "ticket taker" to the sterol party in the gut...it would be too easy if we didn't reuse hyphenated names. But NPC2 runs his leg of the relay before passing the free cholesterol baton to Niemann-Pick C1 (NPC1). If one or both of these runners don't do their job, a horrible disease called Niemann-Pick C Disease results, which has been called "Childhood Alzheimer's" due to its constellation of symptoms that involve severe neurodegeneration.

NPC1 arrives at the plasma membrane and passes the free cholesterol baton to a team member called Aster protein. Maybe you can remember Aster as the "star" of the team, since the term "astral" is related to celestial bodies. But anyway, Aster then transports the free cholesterol to the endoplasmic reticulum, where our anchor leg, the sterol regulatory element binding protein 2 (SREBP2) resides to "bring us home." Prior to the free cholesterol baton arriving, SREBP2 has on his "warm up pants" called SCAP/Insig (a complex involving SREBP cleavage-activating protein and Insulin-induced gene). And if there is enough free cholesterol in the cell, SREBP2 keeps on his sweatpants. But if he needs to "make up lost ground" and free cellular cholesterol is low, he rips off his SCAP/Insig sweatpants (SCAP unbound from Insig activates SREBP2), and races to the Golgi apparatus, our "finish line" of sorts. Subsequently, both nuclear transcription of both HMGCR and LDLR are upregulated. The race has been won!

So, if the cholesterol relay is performed well and the baton is passed appropriately, the cell senses adequate levels of free cholesterol. When levels of free cholesterol are sufficient, the cell will downregulate genes involved in cholesterol synthesis (HMGCR) and cholesterol uptake (LDLR). Conversely, if free cholesterol levels are low, then SREBP2 will increase expression of HMGCR and LDLR.

Understanding some of the issues involved with less-than-ideal racing conditions and proverbial dropping of the free cholesterol baton can help us better make sense of pathologies related to impaired cellular cholesterol homeostasis.

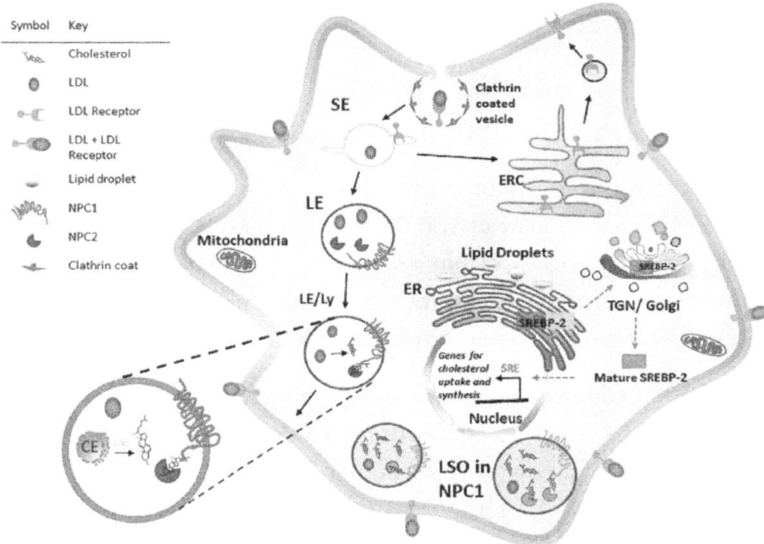

Figure 14: The Intracellular Cholesterol Relay. Just in case you prefer ambiguously labeled diagrams to my metaphors of Olympic sprinters, here's a graphic whose main contribution is to reiterate the complexity of these pathways! Source: Maxfield, F. R., Iaea, D. B., & Pipalia, N. H. (2016). Role of STARD4 and NPC1 in intracellular sterol transport. *Biochemistry and Cell Biology, 94*(6), 499–506. https://doi.org/10.1139/bcb-2015-0154

Lysosomal Acid Lipase Deficiency (Also known as Cholesteryl Ester Storage Disease)

Logically, if cholesteryl ester cannot be properly degraded in the lysosome, that could lead to BIG-TIME problems (and big-time livers and spleens). In the most severe form of lysosomal acid lipase deficiency, called Wolman Disease, these poor kiddos have severe malabsorption (greasy feces), gargantuan livers, and will die within a year without a liver transplant. The less severe form of the disease has a variable presentation. Typically, the patient will have LDL-c levels close to that of someone with Familial Hypercholesterolemia, but it will be accompanied by low HDL-c and elevated liver enzymes. However, the patient will not seem like your typical Standard American Metabolic Disaster, and in-depth histological evaluation will reveal MICROVESICULAR STEATOSIS in the liver along with FOAMY MACROPHAGES. Thankfully, there is enzymatic replacement now available for these individuals which can regulate the intracellular cholesterol relay and make their immune cells a little less frothy.

Diving Deeper: The Role of Saturated Fat

So now that we've discussed the Intracellular Cholesterol Relay, we will be able to answer the age-old question "Why does saturated fat increase LDL cholesterol levels?" which is right up there with historical conundrums involving trees falling in forests and the original order of chickens and eggs.

Remember, cellular cholesterol in the liver is VERY TIGHTLY REGULATED, like Extra-Medium Underarmour on an Extra-Large bro. Any excess of free cellular cholesterol is toxic, so the liver has a few options to avoid this poisonous problem. It can use its cholesterol to make some bile acids, incorporate the cholesterol into lipoproteins, and it can also ESTERIFY the cholesterol. The enzyme that the liver uses to esterify its cholesterol, which involves substituting a fatty acid for the hydroxyl group on the 3rd carbon in the first ring, (see, this is coming "full circle") is called acyl cholesterol acyl transferase 2 (ACAT2).

ACAT2 prefers to use an UNSATURATED FATTY ACID to esterify cholesterol. So, if more unsaturated fatty acids are present, ACAT2 can do its job, esterify the cholesterol, and subsequently the free cholesterol in the plasma membrane decreases. So, SREBP2, the anchor leg in our cholesterol relay, is activated and races to the nucleus to increase LDL receptor expression. So, unsaturated fatty acids tend to decrease LDL-c levels.

Conversely, ACAT2 does NOT prefer to use a saturated fatty acid to esterify cholesterol. Ergo, there is less esterified cholesterol and more free cholesterol in the plasma membrane. The excess free cholesterol means that SREBP2 stays in the endoplasmic reticulum, and LDL receptor activity is downregulated. Less LDL receptor claw-grabbers leads to a logical rise in plasma LDL cholesterol. But not all saturated fats are identical. Shorter chain saturated fats such as lauric and myristic acid tend to have the greatest effect on increasing LDL-c. Conversely, stearic acid, which is the primary saturated fatty acid found in dark chocolate, has a neutral effect on blood cholesterol (and with that, I hopefully just made a bunch of friends)!

So does this mean that we need to avoid saturated fat like the plague? Well, if the ingested saturated fat is coming by way of pizza and Pigs in a Blanket, then by all means. But if you're prioritizing protein and eating real food as part of a reasonable dietary pattern, then I think it probably, in general, doesn't matter a whole lot. However, if you're in a chronically hypercaloric state, it may be a different story...but then again, it always is. That said, if you're an influencer on your soapbox about your perception of the unfair demonization of saturated fat and you're eating sticks of butter on your TikTok channel to "stick it to the man," you may want to re-think your strategy. Because "The Man" or "The System" will just think you're a weirdo, and being gross is a good way to delegitimize your point of view on what may be an otherwise interesting topic of discussion.

Seed Oils

Seed oils? Many view them like that one kid who sat in the back of Biology class who you always kind of avoided. Sometimes he seemed like he could have normal human interactions, but you could never rule out the possibility that he could be a serial killer. And hopefully he grew up to be a successful accountant, but every time you turn on the news you half expect him to be featured in an orange jumpsuit. Although mechanistic plausibility exists regarding lipid peroxidation of seed oils and excess omega-6 in the diet SEEMS nefarious, human trials of linoleic acid consumption (the primary omega-6 fatty acid) are either associated with neutrality or benefit from a cardiovascular standpoint. Studies of dietary intervention are often confounded by many factors, and there are many different seed oils with heterogeneous compositions of omega-3, omega-6, and saturated fatty acids that could potentially exert varying biological effects. I cannot assert, based on the current evidence, that if you are not in a state of overnutrition, that seed oils are harmful. However, no one is forcing you to eat seed oils, and often seed oils are incorporated into many hyper-palatable, ultra-processed foods, which is the real problem. Personally, I just use extra-virgin olive oil, because I feel pretty confident EVOO is a loyal friend who won't end up betraying me someday.

Might as Well Discuss Fiber While We're Here

"Eat more fiber" is often hailed as a dietary axiom...but fiber is actually a rather complicated topic. Because there is insoluble and soluble fiber...and then there are viscous and non-viscous soluble fibers...and there are fermentable and non-fermentable viscous fibers...and all of these fiber types have different functions and stimulate different responses in the gastrointestinal tract. Studying fiber makes you yearn for simpler times when all you knew is that fiber helps you poop.

In general, fiber seems to have some benefit for both blood sugars and lipid levels. It can help lower the glycemic index of a meal, which results in less blood sugar and insulin spikes. Viscous fiber can function sort of like a hybrid bile acid sequestrant/Ezetimibe combo that can have some modest benefit on LDL cholesterol levels. But not everyone has a positive response to fiber; a minority of people see a spike in inflammation levels with increased fiber ingestion, and it can worsen symptoms in certain people with ulcerative colitis and inflammatory bowel disease.

So where does that leave us? Well, I end up landing back at "Prioritize protein, eat real food." Because generally you'll get a reasonable amount of fiber with that approach. And then you can tailor your additional (or subtractional) fiber intake on your individual preferences from there.

Bonus Coverage: Gut Health

Speaking of ~~scams, charlatans, snake oil salesman~~ "Gut Health," countless influencers make confident assertions that if you "heal your gut" then all your problems will dissolve more rapidly than a packet of Athletic Greens in alkaline water. And itinerant entrepreneurs will leverage this into selling prebiotics, probiotics, and pea-biotics (for the Vegans), assuring you that if you "stick with the program," you'll restore your body's proper balance of gut flora and likely eliminate your debt, renew the spark in your marriage, and finally reach the apparent level of euphoria displayed by paid actors in pharmaceutical commercials.

Don't get me wrong...I believe gut health matters...A LOT. I mean, I know firsthand how a bout of amoebic dysentery can completely ruin your life. But in order to rectify what is ABNORMAL, we first must have an understanding of NORMAL. And I don't believe we currently know what the "normal" distribution of gut microbiota looks like...or if there is too much interindividual variability among healthy people to define a "normal" gut microbiome. In order to do this, I believe we would need to ascertain the distribution of gut microbiota in non-insulin resistant young people (by my standards), but would likely need to omit the elite performers (The true reason why the locker room is off-limits to reporters prior to games is because the athletes are destroying the toilets, and cross-country meets are why Porta-Potties are still thriving). Some of the best athletes I've ever competed against have the most irritable of bowels; the dance between the parasympathetic and sympathetic nervous system becomes a frenetic tango for high-level competitors.

But since this is a book on cardiovascular health, I must mention a promising gut-related marker of cardiovascular disease called imidazole propionate (ImP). ImP is produced by gut microbiota in response to the amino acid histidine. When elevated, ImP was correlated with increased risk of subclinical atherosclerosis in the PESA study, and in animal studies was responsible for acceleration of atherosclerosis independent of cholesterol levels.

However, levels of ImP were directly correlated with dysglycemia, elevated hs-CRP, and visceral adiposity...sounds a lot like an impaired Home Security System. So if you merely "Control your insulin, control your life" would ImP vanish as a meaningful risk factor? This remains an unanswered question, so I look forward to future studies in non-insulin resistant populations to determine whether or not this gut metabolite is the "Missing Link" in our evolving understanding of atherosclerotic factors beyond ApoB.

Vitamin D: A Vitamin Deep Dive

The Intracellular Cholesterol Relay is also a nice segue into a discussion about Vitamin D (since sunny days with adequate Vitamin D make for optimal racing conditions). Vitamin D is another one of those soapbox topics where people think that taking colossal quantities will basically lead to immortality and eradicate any vestige of moral delinquency in the process. I would always chuckle when a patient would come to me and say, "I've been a little tired...I think we need to check my Vitamin D." And I would check it, since I'm not a jerk...although I'm skeptical that low Vitamin D is the "smoking gun" when your HbA1c is 13.2 and all of the insects in the Amazonian basis instantly flock to your urine stream every time you enter the bathroom.

So is Vitamin D important in a litany of physiologic functions ranging from immune cell function to calcium homeostasis? Sure. Does it even play a role in cholesterol homeostasis? Actually yes! The short answer is that inadequate levels of Vitamin D can increase cholesterol production and disturb the equilibrium between production and clearance. How does it do this? It's not set in stone, but here's what we think we understand at this point:

- Vitamin D activates the Vitamin D receptor (VDR).
- Adequate VDR signaling leads to SCAP degradation.
- If SCAP is degraded, it doesn't activate SREBP2.
- Decreased SREBP2 leads to decreased cholesterol synthesis and decreased LDL receptor expression.

Conversely, in instances where Vitamin D is deficient, SREBP2 (our relay race "anchor leg") can overcompensate and, instead of just running through the finish line, continues on and runs far beyond the usual end destination, leading to excessive cholesterol production. Additionally, Vitamin D deficiency is a known risk factor for statin-associated myopathic symptoms (SAMS). It would seem that, if your anchor leg is already running too far, giving a statin (which activates SREBP2) would make him run even further off-track into the Great Unknown, potentially leading to some off-target symptoms.

So should we all take Vitamin D? I think it's great to get Vitamin D from sunlight and it's reasonable to supplement if you're deficient. But if you're adequately addressing the elements of your Home Security System, you're probably going to be ok even if your Vitamin D levels are "just normal."

7

BEYOND APOB: TRANSCYTOSIS & ATHEROSCLEROSIS

"I knew exactly what to do. But in a much more real sense, I had no idea what to do."
-Michael Scott, The Office

There is a road in Northern Bolivia named Yungas Road... but it's better known as "Death Road." This highway is precariously poised on the ledges of Andean cliffs and is less than 10 feet wide at many of its hairpin turns. It descends over 11,000 feet through jungles that are generally draped in dense fog, battered by torrential downpours, and prone to capricious landslides. And the road was primarily built by Paraguayan prisoners in the 1930s using primitive tools and discarded rabble. If Death Road is an item on your bucket list, make sure you've checked off all the other destinations first!

There are a variety of problems that can occur with the proverbial highway itself when it comes to development of atherosclerosis. There are rare disorders called mucopolysaccharidoses that result in an impaired ability to construct and repair physiologic highways, so people with mucopolysaccharidoses such as Hurler and Hunter syndrome experience premature vascular disease because it's simply impossible for the ApoB mailmen to deliver their cargo without experiencing a "transcytosis wreckage." (These lysosomal disorders involve various components of the extracellular matrix like glycosaminoglycans, proteoglycans, syndecans, and pretty much every other word that has the suffix "-can").

And there are other less extreme factors that result in lipoproteins transcytosing into the arterial wall and subsequently being retained. We always see more traffic accidents at poorly constructed roundabouts and ill-advised one-way intersections, and disturbances in laminar flow logically can make LDL particles more prone to retention at these sites. Estrogen seems to help "direct traffic" and inhibits LDL transcytosis via the receptor SR-B1. But when estrogen levels precipitously decline in the menopausal transition, unless proper measures are taken, this may result in a "Death Road" type situation when in it comes to vascular and endothelial health! Thankfully, however, both resistance and aerobic exercise PREVENT LDL transcytosis via increasing something called follistatin-like protein-1 (FSTL-1), thus helping "guide traffic." (Weird that exercise keeps coming up as something that's positive for your health).

But there are still more less-understood components involved in ensuring a safe highway that go beyond the realm of traditional cardiovascular risk factors. The mysterious 21.3 region on the short arm of chromosome 9 has long been associated with increased risk for vascular disease, and it appears that this is due to impaired ability to repair damaged endothelium. And curiously, people in the Heart Outcomes Prevention Evaluation (HOPE) trial of the ACE inhibitor Ramipril had reduced cardiovascular events...even if they didn't have high blood pressure! Additionally, modulating the renin-angiotensin-aldosterone system not only reduces blood pressure, but has led to plaque regression in several mechanistic studies.

We could go on, but then I'd have less material for my next book. So I think it's best that we end this section with humility and a quote from the Lipid Legend (and all-around amazing person) Dr. Bill Cromwell:

Although you cannot have atherosclerosis without an ApoB-containing particle infiltrating the arterial intima, "there are other parts of the atherosclerotic process that direct LDL reduction does not always touch...this is a complex process...there is LDL-related risk and there's atherosclerotic risk that may not be LDL-related."

8

AUTOPHAGY

"I've been fasting for 3 days while doing burpees in a sauna...my autophagy must be through the roof!"
-Some YouTube influencer right before dying

Ahh...AUTOPHAGY. Autophagy is another one of those terms that everyone cavalierly throws around without any real understanding of what it means...but we know "autophagy is good." It's sort of the opposite of the word "fascist," which everyone seems to use as an insult, not because we really know what that means, but because "fascism is bad."

The word autophagy literally means "self-eating." And there are many types of autophagy; there is macroautophagy, microautophagy, chaperone-mediated autophagy, mitophagy, tacophagy (just kidding, it's probably not in your body's best interest to eat tacos all the time). But autophagy basically boils down to CELLULAR HOUSEKEEPING. Cells get old and little messes start to accumulate, so it's best to recycle some of the damaged proteins to keep your physiologic abode in a general state of orderliness. And this process involves the lysosome and a swath of cool proteins with names like Beclin-2, GATOR1, and Ragulator.

Anyway, autophagy is the preferred method of housekeeping in contrast to APOPTOSIS. Because when cells become problematically dysfunctional and commit suicide, they leave a swath of pro-inflammatory mediators in their wake.

Essentially, if you have a small mess in your house, you clean things up, take out the garbage, and prevent a ton of junk from accumulating. And this requires a consistently "clean" lifestyle; that's autophagy. Conversely, if big-time messes accumulate and vermin start running roughshod amid the heaps of debris, then you might have to completely set fire to your condemned habitation. That's apoptosis.

So what sort of things promote autophagy? Exercise. Fasting. Not being in a chronic state of overnutrition. Can we measure autophagy? Not really. But we do know that autophagy is regulated by two main nutrient sensors called AMPK and mTOR. AMPK is relatively dominant in states when the cellular AMP to ATP ratio is elevated...this would be when exercising or fasting. Conversely, insulin and nutrient availability are potent activators of mTOR, particularly mTORC1, which is an anabolic pathway.

However, these nutrient sensors are not binary switches that are either "on or off." They are either more relatively dominant or relatively less active depending on the context, and this can even vary depending on the tissue or organ system involved. For instance, you can activate mTORC1 in skeletal muscle simply by performing resistance exercise, although AMPK may be simultaneously dominant in the liver. It's complicated.

Statins and Autophagy
(You thought we were done discussing statins...ha!)

A recent mechanistic study suggests that statins may be regulators of autophagy via activation of FOXO1 (which obviously stands for Forkhead Box Protein O1). If there is a mess in the arterial wall, some intimal housekeeping would seem rather appropriate. However, if FOXO1 is activated in skeletal muscle, mTORC1 is inhibited and mediators of proteostasis such as atrogin-1 (yep, think ATROPHY) are upregulated. Perhaps if you're busy using the Statin Service to clean your house (autophagy), you may not have as much time or energy to use your gym membership (muscle building).

Our bodies are meant to cycle between fasting and fed states. And when we do that, the balance between autophagy and anabolism tends to work out just fine. So should you take your favorite "autophagy activator" like Rapamycin? By all means, you absolutely should if you're a worm indigenous to Easter Island.

But I'm not optimistic that any therapeutic can ever take the place of the following:

- Sleep
- Don't eat crap
- Move
- Cycle between fasting and fed states

Control your insulin, and I think you "control your autophagy" as well.

9

LEAN MASS HYPER-RESPONDERS (LMHRS)

"No one really starts anything new, Mrs. Nemur. Everyone builds on another man's failures. There is nothing really original in science. What each man contributes to the sum of knowledge is what counts."
-Daniel Keyes, Flowers for Algernon

There are a number of individuals who have elected to endorse a ketogenic diet for various reasons. Some have been able to rectify autoimmune issues with this lifestyle, others have ameliorated their mental health, and virtually all of them are prioritizing the mantra, "Control your insulin, control your life."

Many people who adopt a low-carbohydrate diet, particularly if they are overweight, actually see immense improvements in both parameters of glucose metabolism as well as their cholesterol panels. However, in the LMHRs, who typically have a low BMI, there is often a significant spike in LDL cholesterol levels, an HDL cholesterol level that also rises quite profoundly, and a predictably low level of triglycerides. This has formed the basis of the Lipid Energy Model, which posits the following:

- Given the profound degree of dietary carbohydrate restriction, fat is preferentially used as fuel; these folks are continually withdrawing from their "savings account" of fatty acids.
- The liver, which stores glucose as glycogen and normally stores 70-100g of sugar, is also depleted of its glycogen given the profound degree of dietary carbohydrate restriction.
- Insulin levels are quite low, and given that insulin is a "storage hormone" that inhibits lipolysis in fat cells, lipolysis INCREASES and free fatty acids (FFAs) flood back to the liver.
- Free fatty acids determine the rate of VLDL secretion from the liver, so we see increased synthetic rates of these ApoB particles that are going to deliver the fatty acid "mail" to target tissues.
- Given that the mailboxes are not full, the mailmen efficiently deliver the triglyceride mail to the tissues, but since LPL activity is very efficient, there is increased hydrolysis of VLDL to IDL and then to LDL particles. Additionally, the surface free cholesterol (collateral shrapnel from the lipolysis) is also acquired by HDL particles, resulting in elevated LDL-c and HDL-c. But, given the rapid turnover of these previously triglyceride-rich particles, plasma triglycerides remain low.
    - This is the proposed model; however, it is important to remember that most of the "fuel" for oxidative tissues during low insulin states is acquired from liberated free fatty acids rather than lipoprotein-mediated delivery. But anyway, let's move on!

Ok, so there are a lot of moving pieces here and I'm greatly looking forward to the kinetic studies that will help us better understand the adaptive physiologic mechanisms at play. But these core concepts will help guide us as we explore this further:

1. Given that there aren't many "glucose dollar bills" around for energy production, these individuals must continually withdraw from the "fatty acid savings account" to fuel their activities.
2. Given the dearth of dietary carbohydrates, insulin levels will be chronically low in this population.
3. Cells, particularly the cells of the liver, are very sensitive to cholesterol and fatty acid overload; any excess quickly leads to cytotoxicity. So the cells will do what they need to do in order to avoid being drenched in fatty sterol gravy.

With these concepts in mind, here are my Top 5 physiologic musings on what may be going on here:

1. Direct LDL secretion may be having an insulin mimetic anti-lipolytic effect in adipose tissue.
   a. Most LDL particles are typically products of VLDL and IDL hydrolysis...however, there appears to be increased direct LDL secretion in conditions of chronically low triglycerides (this is LDL that isn't first a VLDL). Additionally, given that insulin normally suppresses lipolysis and insulin levels are kept low, it's possible that directly secreted LDL may be "putting the brakes on lipolysis" in fat cells to avoid the liver being drowned in a sea of free fatty acid gravy. Remember, intracellular levels of both cholesterol and fatty acids are tightly regulated. And in experiments of folks with a dietarily-induced rise in LDL-c who have undergone a "re-feed," whether with Oreos or anything else that increases insulin levels, a profound drop in LDL-c has been observed. Insulin clearly has a pivotal role (as it always does)!
2. Put a slightly different way, the low insulin levels will result in increased FFA delivery to the liver. This is

accompanied by a concurrent increase in direct IDL and LDL secretion given the low circulating plasma triglycerides.

   a. This is basically a reiteration of Number 1...the liver is forced to do SOMETHING with all the substrate of fatty acids to mitigate intracellular lipotoxicity... it's just such a key point that I decided to make it Numbers 1 and 2.

3. Also, with the increased FFA delivered to the liver, ACAT2 overexpression results to further minimize the potential lipotoxicity. Esterification of sterols prevents any cholesterol overload, and once esterified, this cholesterol may be packaged into a lipoprotein and re-secreted. But with this ACAT2 overexpression, there will be less cholesterol available for the liver to utilize for its intracellular needs, so it will have to pull the cholesterol from somewhere else. And that leads to a state of INTESTINAL HYPERABSORPTION.
4. In conditions of low insulin, the NPC1L1 ticket-taker in the gut allows more sterols into the party while the ABCG5/G8 bouncers simultaneously "take the day off." This leads to significant hyperabsorption, and some emerging data suggest that Ezetimibe has a much greater effect in reducing LDL cholesterol levels in LMHRs compared to other medications.
   a. There may also be enterocyte-specific downregulation of FXR leading to increased intestinal production of ApoB (as seen in mice where FXR has been knocked out).
   b. If intestinal production of ApoB has, indeed, increased and chylomicron remnants, which carry MUCH more cholesterol per particle and preferentially regulate SREBP2, are being taken up in the liver, the liver will quickly satisfy its intracellular cholesterol demand. Thus, LDL

receptor expression will be inadequate to combat the ongoing fatty flood, perpetuating the hypercholesterolemic state.

c. FXR senses bile acids and normally leads to a decrease in the activity of the ileal bile acid transporter (IBAT). However, if there is decreased intestinal FXR activity, more cholesterol-rich bile acids will be reabsorbed. Indeed, we see a shift to more hydrophobic bile acids which efficiently reabsorb cholesterol in Type 1 diabetes, another condition of low insulin marked by hyperabsorption. Perhaps this is another contributor to the massive LDL-c drop seen in some LMHRs with Ezetimibe usage.

d. Additionally, for someone to display the LMHR phenotype, they may need a "Second Hit" genetically that leads to cholesterol hyperabsorption, such as one or two copies of ApoE4 or mutations in ABCG5/G8. I have a friend who is so shredded that washboards would kill to have abs like him and he has been in ketosis on a strict carnivore diet for the last 3 years. His ApoB is right around 80...the same as it was prior to adopting this dietary regimen. So although leanness may be a prerequisite, it's possible some tendency toward sterol hyperabsorption may also be necessary for the LMHR phenotype to manifest.

5. There may be increased acetoacetyl-CoA synthetase activity reformulating ketone bodies for cholesterol synthesis. Since insulin levels are low, there will be lower activity of transcription factors and enzymes that result in de novo lipogenesis (DNL) such as SREBP1-c and acetyl-CoA carboxylase. So rather than endogenous synthesis of palmitate (DNL), the cytosolic acetyl-CoA will be directed toward cholesterol synthesis.

a. A similar phenomenon results in states of starvation, which is certainly a condition of low insulin.

And there are probably some complexities occurring with the types of fats (saturated vs. unsaturated), the amount of dietary fiber (which will influence absorption rates and potentially other regulators of cholesterol homeostasis), and the ANGPTL family as well, but that chapter and this one are the reasons why we have a Deep End in our Community Pool...enter at your own risk!

Speaking of risk, do these LMHRs have elevated cardiovascular risk despite elevated LDL-c levels? Well, that's a swirling imbroglio of ongoing investigation...some folks, especially those with baseline CAC, seem to have some pretty significant plaque progression while on this dietary regimen. A few seem to be ok so far. The initial results from the KETO-CTA trial didn't strike me as particularly encouraging, but stay tuned as we become privy to more data...that story is far from over and we have much to learn! But at this point, I wouldn't recommend moving to this type of Lipid Neighborhood if you have the option to live elsewhere.

So once again, even though the LMHRs and those who are curious about the underlying mechanisms for the phenomenon have been regarded as "paradigm shifters" in regards to historic dogma surrounding lipids, I feel as confident as ever in the Home Security System and Lipid Neighborhood framework. So here are my recommendations:

- Whatever diet you choose to employ in efforts to "Control your insulin, control your life," don't ignore your Lipid Neighborhood.
- Continue to adhere to the "Got Plaque? Get a CAC!" (and maybe even CCTA) utilization of imaging to better inform you of whether or not there have been

significant break-ins to your arterial abode. If you've been broken into, it appears that you're more likely to experience serial break-ins, and it remains to be seen whether or not certain Lipid Neighborhoods are just "busy but safe" for select individuals who fit this phenotype.

- If you are one of the people who, when adopting a ketogenic diet, experiences an exponential rise in your LDL-c, consider strategies to perhaps live in a slightly safer Lipid Neighborhood. This could include periodic "re-feeds" with some healthy carbohydrates (probably not Oreos...think sweet potatoes or other "real foods") or perhaps a re-evaluation of the types of fats consumed in the diet. Slight adjustments of this nature can maintain the purpose of the diet while not jeopardizing the Lipid Neighborhood.
- If there are compelling medical reasons to not deviate from the strict ketogenic diet, then consider utilizing tools in the lipid-lowering toolbox, particularly if coronary plaque has been identified on imaging. If there are not compelling medical reasons to continue having stratospheric LDL-c levels, consider whether or not this health decision has drifted into the realm of religious tribalism.

I think we can and should Stay Curious while also Staying Reasonable, and even if you disagree with someone on their chosen dietary pattern, please Stay Classy.

Special thanks to the inimitable Jorge Gonzalez for his contributions here...some of these musings are currently unpublished, but stay tuned for about 15 papers on the topic that will soon be available with him as a lead author! I'm grateful to be your "Lipofriend" and we are all your LipoFans.

10

CHOLESTEROL IN THE BRAIN

"Please remember the real me when I cannot remember you."
-Julie White

Dementia is a merciless thief, pilfering the luster from what ought to be golden years while leaving broken hearts and shattered dreams in its unforgiving wake. There's a massive difference between existing and truly living. Having just lost my grandmother to Alzheimer's Disease, I am particularly passionate about this topic, and I believe that despite the absurd complexity of lipids in the brain, I can hopefully offer some key takeaways from my several-hundred-page dissertation on the topic. There is significant overlap between risk factors for cardiovascular disease and neurodegeneration, and while the generalization that "whatever helps the heart is good for the brain" is mostly accurate, there are many enigmatic variables that remain under investigation. Despite these unknowns, I believe I can not only help you start to view dementia, specifically the Alzheimer's type, through a lipid-centric lens, but impart hope for the future as we all seek to find a solution or combination of approaches to mitigate the ravages of this horrible disease.

Healthy Heart, Healthy Brain...Is It That Simple?

In general, what's good for the heart is good for the brain. Regular exercise is associated with a 45% decreased risk of Alzheimer's disease, and those with the highest cardiorespiratory fitness have the lowest incidence of dementia. Conversely, those with the highest CAC scores in MESA had the highest risk of dementia, and those with ASCVD in midlife from the UK BioBank had 29% increased risk of Alzheimer's. Additionally, obesity, diabetes, and hyperinsulinemia all are strongly associated with cognitive decline. But since it's the brain, there's a little more to the story!

Most people have heard of the *APOE* genotype as the number one genetic risk factor for Alzheimer's disease. You inherit one *APOE* copy from each parent, and about 75% of people have 2 copies of *APOE3*. However, if you have one copy of *APOE4*, it increases your risk of Alzheimer's by three to fourfold, and if you have 2 copies of *APOE4*, you may be about 12 times more likely to develop Alzheimer's. This has recently garnered significant public attention, since the actor Chris Hemsworth, notorious for his role as Thor (APOE-Thor, perhaps)? has the *APOE4/4* genotype.

But I don't believe that even those like Chris are necessarily destined for dementia despite their genetic susceptibility. I believe that if the appropriate lifestyle measures are taken across the lifespan to maintain a virtually pristine Home Security System, then the downstream perturbations in cholesterol regulation will be abrogated. Alois Alzheimer himself first noted toxic lipid droplets in the brains of those with cognitive impairment, and in my view, Alzheimer's, as well as many neurodegenerative diseases, are really lipid disorders. (I mean, when you're a hammer everything looks like a nail, but particularly when conditions of aberrant lipid transport like Niemann-Pick C

Disease lead to "Childhood Alzheimer's," I stand by it). I view the abnormal accumulation of the amyloid beta protein and the subsequent tau hyperphosphorylation that characterize Alzheimer's as downstream consequences of impaired cholesterol homeostasis. Your genetics give you more or less margin for error, but I believe if you never let fires start, you don't have to worry about a defective fire department.

Cholesterol in the brain is wildly different and kept separate from what is going on in the peripheral circulation. The half-life of cholesterol in the brain is 6 months to 5 years, there are no ApoB mailmen, and instead the main "mailman" is an HDL-like character that is mainly an ApoE particle.

Normally in the brain, glial cells called astrocytes make cholesterol, the cholesterol is exported into an ApoE HDL, and then the ApoE HDL delivers the cholesterol to the neuron, where it serves critical roles in a myriad of processes. Remember, making cholesterol is energetically expensive, and it's ideal for the neuron to use its energy to basically "run the show" rather than worrying about synthesizing cholesterol. And then if there is too much cholesterol around, the neuron can get rid of the excess by turning it into something called 24s-hydroxycholesterol. All is well.

But without getting too granular, there are 3 consistent categories of cholesterol disturbances in the brains of those with Alzheimer's Disease:

1. **Impaired cholesterol transport**
   a. This is a big part of the ApoE story, as ApoE4 HDL-like particles are not as efficient at picking up the cholesterol for subsequent delivery. And if transport is inefficient, then cholesterol accumulates where it doesn't belong.
2. **Impaired cholesterol elimination**

   a. If cholesterol is accumulating and not being eliminated, it leads to neuroinflammation.
3. **Impaired cholesterol synthesis**
   a. The toxic cholesterol metabolites that have accumulated where they don't belong negatively feedback on cholesterol production, further exacerbating the vicious cycle.

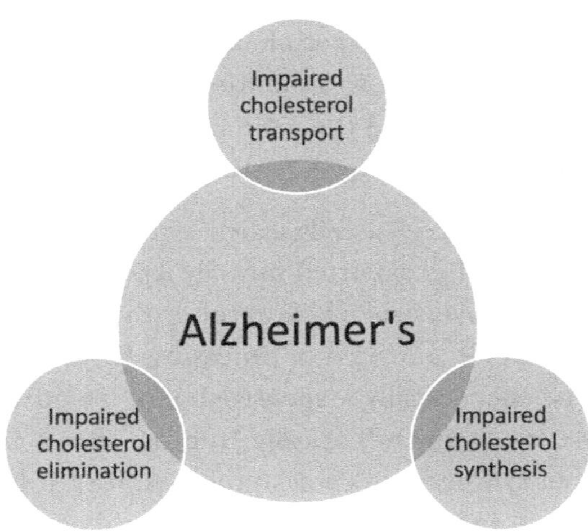

Figure 12: Cholesterol Disturbances in the Alzheimer's Brain

ApoE4 particles are like "easily distractable" members of a busy office, and instead of doing their jobs of cholesterol transport, they often leave messes. The neurons are the higher-ranking executives who depend on proper memos being delivered to them, but if the ApoE4 particles never get them the messages, problems ensue. The microglia, which are the brain's inflammatory cells, get annoyed with the ApoE4 particles and propagate an inflammatory response. And then the neurons start making their own ApoE to try to compensate for what the ApoE4 HDL should have been doing; when neurons are forced to perform the job of some other cell, you're asking for burnout. And then eventually everything shuts down.

And that's what we consistently see in the Alzheimer's brain: impaired cholesterol transport, impaired cholesterol elimination, and decreased cholesterol synthesis. And there are SO MANY lipid players involved in the regulation of this process beyond ApoE, including PCSK9, ApoA-1, and the LDL receptor family. For instance, PCSK9 is particularly promiscuous, binding to many different protein partners in the brain. PCSK9 is consistently elevated in those with Alzheimer's as well as in *APOE4* carriers, but we need to determine whether or not it is a bystander in the process or an actual promoter of disease progression. Conversely, ApoA-1 deficiency may be a risk factor for Alzheimer's (and what increases ApoA-1...yep, exercise)! ApoA-1 seems to help the microglia perform their cellular housekeeping duties more effectively, and any time exercise seems to be the right answer, I feel like the retrograde hypothesis has at least some degree of plausibility. However, we need to better understand the role of all the various players that are associated with more or less susceptibility to the disease process.

But what is exciting to me is that biomarkers to identify Alzheimer's in early stages are IMPROVING BY THE DAY. And even though the complexity of brain lipids is ridiculous, I believe that the questions all of us in this field have proposed ARE KNOWABLE with further research. And it may be quixotic, but I believe that metabolic and lipid-oriented cocktails will eventually be a critical component of a proactive and individualized regimen for people who are identified as having "subclinical Alzheimer's." And I firmly believe that we can have a future in which the vast extent of neurodegenerative disease becomes a distant memory.

DEEP DIVE: BDNF and Cholesterol in the Brain

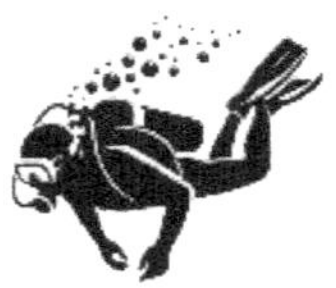

We know that exercise, through many diverse mechanisms, is unequivocally beneficial for preserving cognitive function across the lifespan. And anyone who has ever listened to a Rhonda Patrick podcast is probably aware that one of the putative ways in which exercise ameliorates brain health is via stimulating production of brain-derived neurotrophic factor, or BDNF. The name itself suggests it's a key player in neuronal development and synaptic function, but the real intrigue lies in BDNF's role in brain cholesterol homeostasis.

As stated previously, the typical way by which neurons acquire cholesterol is via astrocytic delivery. However, BDNF decreases cholesterol uptake by the neuron...at first blush, that seems problematic! But, BDNF also stimulates NEURONAL CHOLESTEROL SYNTHESIS in a region of the neuron called the lipid raft region. This region, which contains many cholesterol-loving caveolin proteins, functions as a platform on which cell signaling, transduction, and neurotransmission take place. Without adequate amounts of cholesterol in these lipid rafts, your neurons have trouble "staying afloat" with all the cellular processes they are attempting to orchestrate.

So how do we make sense of this? Well, it's currently in the theoretical realm, but I believe that exercise "gives the ApoE delivery guys" a break. Typically, the neuron receives its cholesterol from the ApoE particles, but exercise allows the neuron to synthesize its own cholesterol. This may have particularly important implications for those with one or two copies of ApoE4, as the inefficiency and distractability of the ApoE4 mailmen may be mitigated by the direct BDNF-mediated neuronal cholesterol production. Similar to how exercise allows skeletal muscle to take up glucose without the need of insulin, I believe that exercise may allow the neuron to acquire its critical cholesterol content without depending on a potentially faulty delivery system. And, over time, this may very well attenuate the lipotoxicities that could otherwise occur in the central nervous system, particularly in those with ApoE4.

THE GRAND CONCLUSION

"Come to Me, all you who are weary and heavy-laden, and I will give you rest."
-Matthew 11:28

I hope you've enjoyed exploring the Home Security System and Lipid Neighborhood. I hope that it has equipped you with a basic framework to help you and your loved ones avoid heart attacks, strokes, and dementia. I hope all the anthropomorphisms and analogies have helped you understand the fascinating role of cholesterol and lipoproteins in the human machine. And I hope that amidst all the walking with kings, some semblance of common touch was retained so that you could smile and perhaps even chuckle a time or two along the way.

But I believe that the most profound analogy when it comes to metabolic health is, in fact, a spiritual one, and I think a story from one of my patients best illustrates this concept. I had a patient who came to me with sky-high blood sugars and a HbA1c of 12.6 (anything over 6.5 is diabetes...really on the struggle bus here). So I did what I could to optimize her medications, obtained a continuous glucose monitor for her, and gave her the Josh Reversal of Diabetes Dietary Menu that had worked for numerous others in her situation. I felt pretty good about things.

After a few months, she was doing slightly better, and her HbA1c was down to 9.8...progress, but certainly not ideal by any means. Her morning blood sugars were stratospheric, and I checked for some unusual causes of "Type 1.5" diabetes, which she didn't have. I asked her about her diet, and she insisted she was very strict about it, so I requested she keep a dietary journal until I saw her again.

The next time I saw her, her blood sugars had remained dizzyingly high and she had made absolutely no progress. But the crazy thing was she had even started going to the gym, had continued the prescribed dietary regimen, and was dutifully logging her food intake. Additionally, she was on ALL the magic sauce of medications, and we just weren't getting anywhere. She was understandably frustrated, and my initial thoughts were to go zebra-hunting for previously undiscovered causes of diabetes...but then I asked her, "Do you have sleep apnea?" She didn't think so, but she didn't know, and I sent her for a sleep study. Lo and behold, she had SEVERE sleep apnea, and after getting her continuous positive airway pressure (CPAP) device, at her 3-month follow-up appointment her HbA1c was 5.8. Her body had been stressed when it should have been at rest, but once that was rectified, she was well on her way to restoring her metabolic health.

And that, to me, was such a powerful real-life example of the importance of REST. You can meticulously DO all the right things in regards to diet, exercise, and even employ the very best medications at the same time...but without sleep, you're never going to get anywhere.

And sleep is a funny thing, since it's PASSIVE. You can't say, "I'm going to try REALLY HARD to get a good night's sleep."

You stay awake all night with that approach. How do you "get good sleep?" You lay down and just let go.

And for all of us, our collective human problem is that we're all a bunch of imperfect people. We don't need to go trying to figure out some weird cause of all our existential struggles...the problem is sin. The omnipotent Creator of the universe sets an impossible standard of perfection, and even though you and I might not be "as bad as Hitler" or some other evil person, we're still messed up. And you can try to be an altruistic person and do some good things, fill your mind with positive, motivational, spiritual thoughts, and perhaps even genuflect at the altar of academia. But if you first aren't RESTING and trusting in the only One who has the antidote for your sin condition, it's like trying to diet and exercise with severe sleep apnea. You're exhausting yourself and locked in a losing battle.

But that's when you let go. You realize that you can't save yourself and attain that impossible perfect standard that would satisfy the justice of a holy and supreme deity. But when you realize that, despite your sin condition, Jesus Christ lived the sinless life you and I never could, died the criminal's death on the cross that you and I deserved, and then defeated the power of sin and death by rising again, all you have to do is just believe. He says, "Come to Me, all you who are weary and heavy laden, and I will give you rest." Rest from the perpetual struggle. Rest for your soul.

And then when you do place your trust in the One who overcame the power of death, then you will continually fill your mind with wonderful and beautiful things and DO things like show kindness to others while exuding love, joy, peace, and patience. Once you're getting that all-important rest, the other features of a spiritually healthy person will follow naturally. Just as the intersection of metabolic pathways is infinitely complicated, the solution is beautifully simple. Sleep. Move. Put quality fuel in the machine. Love with all you've got. And repeat every day until God takes you home. And instead of being crushed under the pressure of obligatory burdens, life becomes an overwhelming blessing and an exciting adventure in which we can embrace the immense privilege of exquisitely beautiful forays into topics such as cholesterol homeostasis!

And because I don't know the future, but I know the One who holds it, I know I have fail-proof Home Security...not because of anything I did, but because of what He has already done. And I know my ultimate Neighborhood is a heavenly one, so I can truly rest in peace when all is said and done.

EPILOGUE

Everyone loves a good redemption story...from Dickens' *Tale of Two Cities* to Dostoevsky's *Crime and Punishment* to ~~Lance Armstrong,~~ it's human nature to "root for the underdog" and to desire atonement for past wrongs. And my favorite redemption story is that of the apostle Peter in John 21.

Peter was a successful fisherman before Jesus called him to be his disciple. And Peter's life was characterized by both stratospheric heights and colossal failures of subterranean proportions. He briefly became the first regular guy ever to walk on water...and then had to rely on Jesus to save him from drowning when his faith failed him. He boldly declared Jesus to be the Messiah in Matthew 16...then a few verses later was rebuked for speaking on behalf of Satan. He was privy to a foreshadowing of the glories of Heaven on the Mount of Transfiguration...and then couldn't stay awake when Jesus' only command was to keep his eyes open.

On numerous occasions, Peter had proven that the entrance to his mouth was demonstrably foot-shaped, and he even brashly claimed that he would die for Jesus. But when Jesus was in his darkest hour, as He was being spat upon, mocked, beaten, and scourged before his crucifixion, Peter denied that he even knew Jesus. Not once. Not twice. But three times.

And at that point, Peter knew he had failed. He had REALLY wanted to be a disciple of Jesus. He had REALLY wanted to demonstrate that he was worthy of this high calling. But he knew that his resume was sorely lacking. He knew that he deserved to be "cut from the team." And he knew that whatever Jesus was looking for in a disciple, it surely wasn't somebody like him.

But at least he was good at fishing...or so he thought. But when he tried to return to his old occupation, he spent all night long out on the lake with his buddies...and caught nothing. This is sort of like selling Pest Control door to door for commission only...the only thing I ever got when I did that job for a week was a brutal farmer's tan and a few granola bars from people who felt bad for me...pretty depressing.

And then Jesus showed up on the shore. "You guys haven't caught anything, have you?" the omniscient Lord of the Universe asked rhetorically. (This had to be aggravating...sort of like when Uncle Tony used to ask you how your football game went when he knew full-well that your team got demolished 54-0). "Why don't you try the other side of the boat?" Jesus suggested, as if somehow the fish in the Sea of Galilee had chiral preferences. And, of course, they instantly caught 153 fish. Realizing that Jesus had orchestrated this miraculous haul, Peter impulsively splashed towards the shore, leaving his friends to laboriously lug the catch to shore. Despite his failures, all he ever wanted was to be with Jesus.

And then Jesus asked Peter a simple question. "Peter, do you love me?" Three times, Jesus asked Peter that question...the same number of times Peter had denied that he even knew Jesus several days prior. And the first two times, the Greek word that Jesus used for love was *agape*, which means unconditional love...

the type of love that Jesus Himself had demonstrated to the world. Peter knew that his love didn't measure up, so he answered, "Well, yeah I *fileo* you (not a reference to a longitudinal trout cutlet, but the Greek word meaning "brotherly affection"). The third time, Jesus asked Peter, "Do you even *fileo* me?" Peter was truly shattered. This once-proud bombastic brute, formerly bursting with bravado, had been brought to his knees. And that's exactly where he needed to be. Because Peter had to learn that Jesus was the one who was not only in control of the fish in the sea, but in control of the type of fishing that Peter would be doing the rest of his life. And that impulsive failure of a fisherman, his cowardice changed to courage by the transforming love of Christ, became the Rock upon which the church was built. He became a Fisher of Men.

In many ways, I feel a lot like Peter. I've had the immense privilege of dipping my toe in many waters and plumbing the depths of scientific discovery. I relish the Deep Dives of exploring previously uncharted biochemical territories, and sometimes I become so entranced that I don't even want to come up for air. I've achieved some measure of success in these proverbial fishing expeditions by earthly standards. But ultimately, I believe that God has also called me to be a Fisher of Men. Questions such as, "Have you checked your Lp(a)?" and "Have you gotten a CAC?" are pretty important when it comes to your heart health. But ultimately, the most important question regarding your eternal heart health is the same question Jesus asked Peter: "Do you love me?"

There have been times in my life that I've tried to "go back to fishing." I know I haven't loved Jesus with the perfect love with which He has loved me. I've failed over and over again, and I've felt unworthy to be called His disciple. But I know that despite my imperfections, God doesn't leave projects unfinished. And I take solace in the fact that He will never, ever give up on me.

So do I love lipids? Of course. Do I love people? Absolutely. And do I love Jesus? Because He first loved me, I do. And my prayer is that you come to know His unconditional love and the accompanying peace that surpasses understanding as well.

FREQUENTLY ASKED QUESTIONS

1. **How tall are you?**
   - 5'10 and ¾, but generally 5'11" or greater if you count my hair.
2. **How much do you weigh?**
   - Inappropriately personal question. But let's just say it's somewhere between an adult capybara and a professional marathon runner.
3. **Can you dunk a basketball?**
   - At this stage in the game, I'm a holy terror on 8-foot rims. And if I've gotten about 10 hours of sleep, I'm not sore from Crossfit, the stars are perfectly aligned, and you give me about 30-45 minutes to warm up, I can still dunk a tennis ball on a 10-foot hoop...by the time this book is published that may have changed, however.
4. **What is your favorite Pokémon?**
   - Diglett, obviously.
5. **What are your thoughts on cold tubs/cold plunges for metabolic health?**
   - It actually can "beige" your fat cells. You increase the mitochondrial content in your white fat via

induction of something called PGC1-α, since your body needs to make a survival-istic adaptation to stay warm. The increased mitochondrial content makes your fat more brown. And if mitochondria aren't generating ATP, they are "uncoupled" and this generates a waste product in the form of heat. So in this instance, inefficiency in fat is actually useful, whereas mitochondrial inefficiency in your skeletal muscle is clearly a bad thing. But I personally hate the cold...because I like it warm.

6. **What are your thoughts on sauna?**
   - The data demonstrating association between sauna use and decreased risk of Alzheimer's is quite impressive, and it activates some beneficial metabolic pathways via various heat shock proteins. I think the most significant barrier is the inevitable presence of an unashamedly and unambiguously nude gentleman intent on telling you his life story upon entry into the sauna. And that guy is never young, so buckle up.
7. **Help! My doctor told me I have chronic kidney disease! I just finished first in my age group in a local Triathlon, I deadlift 3x my body weight, and I volunteer at the local humane society...how is this even possible?! Also my doctor told me reduce my protein intake...I already feel weaker!**
   - If you are supplementing with creatine, you can have an artificially decreased GFR because the typical estimation of GFR is based on creatinine clearance. This is also influenced by muscle mass. Creatinine is a byproduct of the phosphocreatine reaction, and since you're supplementing with creatine, you will be providing more substrate for the reaction to occur. This does NOT mean that you have kidney damage. But just to make sure, this is where you

request a lab called cystatin c, which is not influenced by creatine usage or muscle mass. And almost every time I've checked this in a concerned, athletic creatine user, it's been 100% normal. If that's the case, keep taking your creatine and keep prioritizing protein.

8. **You didn't mention Lp-PLA2, polygenic risk scores, OxPL-ApoB, desmosterolosis, lipoprotein glomerulopathy, or Smith-Lemli-Opitz Syndrome...what's wrong with you? Aren't you a lipid specialist?**
    - I never intended this book to be exhaustive OR exhausting.
9. **You still didn't talk about homocysteine...what gives?**
    - Homocysteine is an interesting biomarker and is associated with everything from strokes to dementia...but when you have a patient who recently had her HbA1c and homocysteine checked by another "holistic provider" and both numbers were 12.8...and the only recommendation given by this practitioner was to take a complex of methylated B-vitamins...well, forgive me for not fixating on her C677T heterozygosity in the MTHFR gene. But take heart! I fully intend on getting into the deep weeds on homocysteine in a future book on nutrition and supplements...maybe the title will be "Supp, Y'all?" and I'll leverage my hip-hop background to rap about methylation.
10. **What about intermittent fasting?**
    - The trifecta of factors to consider when discussing diet are what you eat (macronutrient distribution), how much you eat (caloric intake), and when you eat. If the "when," of intermittent fasting or time-restricted feeding can help you address the critical

"what" and "how much" components, then it can be a useful tool.

11. **How do you feel about the concept of "Primordial Prevention?"**
    - Fatty streaks in blood vessels, the earliest signs of atherosclerosis, were found in stillborn babies of mothers with Familial Hypercholesterolemia. Autopsies of young soldiers who paid the ultimate sacrifice in battle demonstrated similar pathology. And the PDAY study showed both fatty streaks and plaques in the vasculature of individuals aged 15 to 34. Atherosclerosis can potentially start at birth, so a recent group of passionate preventers has coined the term Primordial Prevention. But what does this really mean? Should we statinize babies the moment they take their first steps? Rather than teach infants the ABCs, should we be first teaching them the letters L-D-L? I think that sometimes people misconstrue the message as extreme. I think it simply means we emphasize early identification of the various factors that can result in atherosclerosis rather than taking a laissez-faire approach to coronary disease. And I don't think there's anything wrong with that.
12. **Why didn't you discuss the Women's Health Initiative to a greater extent? And what about initiating HRT in the perimenopausal period?**
    - Others such as Avrum Bluming and Carol Tavris have written about the WHI rather eloquently, and if you're more of a Social Media person, Dr. Heather Hirsch has some quality content on the topic as well. Regardless, it's very important that you find a practitioner who "gets it" and, more importantly, understands YOU when it comes to HRT.
13. **What are your thoughts on coffee?**

  - Coffee, also known as the Elixir of Life, generally has very little impact on cholesterol metrics. However, unfiltered coffee, due to its elevated diterpene content, can actually raise LDL-c levels. So just filter your coffee and you can continue to reap coffee's host of benefits without any fear of jeopardizing your Lipid Neighborhood. Because without coffee, you may very well not have the will to do anything productive when it comes to reinforcing your Home Security System...I've done case studies on myself, and without it I'm about as useless as decaf.

14. **What supplements do you take?**
    - Magnesium and creatine.
15. **What do you do for exercise?**
    - Everything. I will "run socially" if someone wants to go out and jog, but mainly you'll find me lifting, sprinting, jumping, playing racquetball, basketball, soccer, Ultimate Frisbee, coaching high school cross country, and embarrassing myself at my daughter's gymnastics class...definitely past my prime, but enjoying the battle against inevitable decline.
16. **Speaking of exercise, do you have any thoughts on VO2 max?**
    - There has recently been quite the emphasis on VO2 max as a useful metric in regards to cardiovascular mortality. And this isn't real surprising...when you play the game "Who Is More Likely to Die?" you don't usually pick the Olympic cross-country skier over the diabetic pirate with one leg. However, I think that if you emphasize PERFORMANCE, you probably don't really need to worry about getting your VO2 max tested...those that were able to achieve 14 metabolic equivalents (METs) were 4 times more likely to not die compared to those in the lowest 20% of cardiorespiratory fitness in a study

of over 750,000 people followed over a decade. 14 METs is about a 7-minute mile, so if you can target a high level of aerobic performance based on your orthopedic status, you'll probably be feeling pretty decent about the future.

17. **How do you feel about the concept of "cumulative exposure to elevated levels of atherogenic lipoproteins" being compared to long-term cigarette smoking?**
    - It's a popular and trendy thing to compare "pack years" of smoking to "plaque years" of exposure to high LDL-c levels. Not everyone who smokes gets lung cancer, even though it has proven causal to lung cancer pathogenesis, and many smokers predictably do get lung cancer. However, cancer or not, smoking causes unequivocal damage to one's healthspan and functional status. High LDL-c (like heterozygous familial hypercholesterolemia) often leads to atherosclerosis, but not always. However, in contrast to smoking, some of these folks seem to have no decrement in healthspan due to these high LDL-c levels, which should encourage us to research these situations further. So although the "pack years and plaque years" is a pithy catchphrase, I'm sticking with my Home Security System and Lipid Neighborhood framework.

APPENDIX A

A Brief History of Cholesterol

As I was considering why this section would be called an "Appendix," I came to an epiphany; although you don't NEED an appendix, your life is probably better if you have one. So here you go!

The history of drug development is fraught with serendipity, hilarity, and sometimes abject failure. For instance, one of the first attempts at a weight-loss drug was dinitrophenol (DNP), a mitochondrial uncoupling agent found in TNT munitions factories. A bunch of the workers were unintentionally losing weight, so pharma was hoping DNP could explode onto the scene as an effective way to help fit into those trendy corsets...unfortunately, DNP is a little TOO much like dynamite and everyone pretty much died of malignant hyperthermia.

However, one of the MOST successful drug classes of all time, the GLP-1 receptor agonists, came about when some scientists were playing around with lizard spit. Apparently when gila monsters, which are basically miniature Komodo dragons, bite you, it makes your pancreas swell, but if you don't die it improves your blood sugars. And because of that, we find ourselves firmly planted in the "Age of Ozempic." This is also why we encourage kids to play in the backyard and demonstrate a healthy curiosity that teeters right on the edge of lethality...for science!

The discovery of cholesterol wasn't quite as dramatic; no reptilian saliva was involved and no one exploded, but it did involve a Frenchman and some gallstones. Most gallstones are cholesterol-rich, and Francois Poulletier de la Salle first made this observation in 1769 (you may know that a *cholecystectomy* is when you get your gall bladder removed, and the gall bladder stores bile. *Chole* is the Greek word for bile). Words are fun!

Time went on, and in the early 20th century some guys started stuffing rabbits with absurd quantities of human food, including meat and eggs, and ended up inducing a ton of plaques in their arteries. (America has since tried a similar strategy with people, except with Cheetos, Twinkies, and Mountain Dew, and has been diabolically successful in achieving the same outcome). A buddy of Joseph Stalin named Nikolai Anichkov also got involved with rabbit stuffing, specifically with cholesterol, and it was theorized that this phenomenon of atherosclerosis was cholesterol-dependent. This was accepted as a reasonable assertion...although I'd say the more straightforward conclusion is that you get raging heart disease when you feed herbivores a bunch of food unsuitable for their native physiology.

One of the pioneers in discovery of LIPOPROTEINS was a guy named John Gofman. Interestingly, Gofman had been in cahoots with Oppenheimer on the Manhattan Project during World War II. Plagued by existential guilt after the develop- ment of the atomic bomb, he instead shifted his focus to lipids; he sought redemption through medical research. By using an ultracentrifuge to better characterize the densities of various lipoproteins, he achieved a "cholesterol catharsis" of sorts and left an enduring gift to humanity, earning the title "Father of Clinical Lipidology." (Parents, when your kids are sent to the principal's office, leverage this as an opportunity to channel their penance into learning about cholesterol).

Some guys like Ancel Keys determined that blood levels of cholesterol were associated with cardiovascular disease, so some catastrophic attempts along the lines of DNP were made to lower cholesterol. Thyroid hormone lowers cholesterol...so some people thought giving extra thyroid hormone was a good idea; this was a quick recipe for atrial fibrillation and/or death. Women seem to get less heart disease than men, at least for a while, so some other people thought giving estrogen to men was a good idea. (Spoiler: didn't work). And some heavy-duty antibiotics called aminoglycosides also incidentally lower cholesterol... so that was tried as well.

And a bunch of other stuff happened until Michael Jackson's 1982 *Thriller* album forever changed the trajectory of pop culture and music videos...oh yeah, and statins...they were being developed at the same time. And the rest is history!

APPENDIX B

B for Board Exam! The table below contains a few select pathologies that frequently pop up on Lipid Boards.

Condition	Characteristics	Comments
Tangier Disease	Defect in ABCA1 HDL-c <5 Orange tonsils, hepatosplenomegaly, peripheral neuropathy Autosomal recessive	Tangier-orange Tonsils with HDL levels in the Toilet
Familial Hypoalphalipoproteinemia	Mutation in APOA1 Non-existent HDL-c AND ApoA-1 Premature and accelerated atherosclerosis Autosomal Dominant	Big-time bummer
Familial LCAT Deficiency and Fish Eye Disease	HDL-c <10 Progressive kidney disease and coronary disease Hemolytic anemia and corneal opacities Presence of Lipoprotein X	When you can't esterify HDL-c, you can't "c" straight (corneal opacities), you get CKD, and you get CAD. Less severe form you just look like a fish

	Autosomal Recessive	
ApoA-1 Milano	Super low HDL-c, but with SUPERPOWERS No cardiovascular disease despite low HDL-c	When Lil Jon and the East Side Boyz produced the song "Get Low" they were probably referring to this
Abetalipoproteinemia and Chylomicron Retention Disease (CMRD)	Genetic defect in MTTP Undetectable ApoB Malabsorption, fat soluble vitamin deficiency, neurological issues, retinitis pigmentosa Autosomal Recessive	Abetalipoproteinemia-no ApoB mailmen, no Absorption, ADEK deficiency, spinocerebellar Ataxia CMRD-same phenotype but due to defect in SAR1B GTPase
Hypobetalipoproteinemia	Truncated ApoB-100 variants Plasma ApoB <40 mg/dL Generally asymptomatic, maybe some fatty liver Low risk of CAD	Other variants include PCSK9 and ANGPTL3 loss-of-function. ANGTL3 LOF is characterized by low LDL-c and low HDL-c and may be called Familial Combined Hypolipidemia

		Low lifetime risk of CAD across the board
Cerebrotendinous Xanthomatosis (CTX)	Defect in CYP27A1 (27-hydroxylase) Toxic accumulation of cholestanol and bile alcohols Diarrhea, tendinous xanthomas, foot deformities, neurologic issues, cataracts Treatment: chenodeoxycholic acid Autosomal Recessive	Since FXR regulates bile homeostasis, dysregulation can lead to catarax, xanthomas, ataxia, and it's like you're on a laxative if you have CTX
Lysosomal Acid Lipase Deficiency (Cholesteryl Ester Storage Disease)	LDL-c levels similar to HeFH (190 or greater) but with low HDL-c and elevated LFTs Microvesicular hepatic steatosis and foamy macrophages Most severe form is Wolman Disease, which	Labs look like a hybrid of fatty liver/metabolic syndrome/familial hypercholesterolemia

	needs liver transplant. Less severe-enzymatic replacement Autosomal Recessive	
Type III Dysbetalipoproteinemi a	Remnant lipoprotein disease Accelerated atherosclerosis, palmar xanthomas High total cholesterol and high triglycerides with normal ApoB Usually E2/E2 genotype with a "Second Hit" of insulin resistance, alcohol, or medications that impair clearance of triglyceride rich lipoproteins	Total cholesterol/ApoB ratio >6.2 with Triglyceride/ApoB ratio <10

APPENDIX E

EVEN MORE APOLIPOPROTEINS!

What happened to Appendices C and D, you ask? Didn't need them!

Apolipoprotein	**Characteristics**	**Comments**
ApoA2 and ApoA3	ApoA2: 2nd most abundant protein on HDL ApoA3: Doesn't exist, apparently	Like Nelly said, "2 is not a winner, and 3 nobody remembers"
ApoA4	Produced in response to high-fat feeding May have a role in reducing inflammatory bowel disease, eosinophilic conditions, and platelet aggregation	Could have a role in the anecdotally positive response of certain individuals with ulcerative colitis/Crohn's disease to a ketogenic diet
ApoD	Associated with arachidonic acid; likely plays a role in modulating oxidative stress	Generally just used as the subject of dirty jokes by lipidologists
ApoF	An inhibitory protein of CETP; activity is inversely correlated with triglyceride levels and CETP activity	When LDL-c is high, ApoF activity is high. When triglyceride levels are high, ApoF activity is low.

ApoH	Associated with hypercoagulable states, some autoimmune conditions, and Lp(a)	Also known as beta-2 glycoprotein
ApoL1	Has anti-trypanosoma activity	When it's not swatting away tsetse flies, it may be giving people CKD in those of African descent
ApoJ	Potentially significant in amyloid clearance/Alzheimer's disease, also known as clusterin	My name starts with J and at times, I also feel poorly understood
ApoM	Protein on HDL particles that integrates sphingosine-1 phosphate into HDL Helps pre-beta HDL develop and important in efflux capacity	An intriguing apolipoprotein that likely is important in HDL functionality
ApoO	A couple of articles showed elevations of whatever this is in diabetics	Pretty sure that this one never really caught on since it looks like "Apoo"

APPENDIX T

T for "Tube" (just because you needed one more ridiculous story from my High School Experience).

When I was in High School, I was actually considered "cool." I had earned the title "Mr. Meridian High School" and was also elected Student Body President. I held this position about half the year until I said something stupid with an open microphone in front of the entire school and was subsequently removed from office (another good story for the next book I write).

Early during my Senior Year, I was helping my teacher mount an oversized World Map on the wall of my first period class. This map had nothing to offer me, as I had already memorized all those nations and their capitals back in second grade, but I was struck by the potential of the cylindrical unit in which the map had previously been stored. My first thought was to employ this tube as a striking implement for Hallway Baseball, but the tube's girth prohibited a natural swing. So instead, I spray-painted the cylinder blue and in fluorescent yellow bubble letters wrote "TUBE" on the vessel.

I then proceeded to tell everyone that this tube was going to symbolize our ascendancy to the pinnacle of athletic and academic success during our school year. Obviously this outrageous, borderline irrational statement was immediately dismissed as doggerel, right? WRONG! The "MERIDIAN HIGH SCHOOL TUBE" quickly displaced the Warrior as our unofficial mascot, was paraded proudly at football games, and became a prominent fixture at all major school events. A tube labeled "tube."

So when some "medical expert" mandates a policy or some guy with a tube convincingly makes a charismatic statement, you probably ought to read the proverbial nutrition facts prior to drinking the Kool-aid. Unless, of course, your one goal is to get promoted at your company or be Resident of the Year...then by all means imbibe freely. You may just get the next Breakfast of Champions award while you're at it.

REFERENCE ROADMAP

Since I didn't want to compromise the readability of the book, I decided to not litter the manuscript with a thousand footnotes and superscripted numerical references (that's what my PhD dissertation was for, and no one reads that unless they're struggling with insomnia). So I felt the most logical way to reference the cited material was to first briefly notate the publication chapter by chapter in general order of appearance, and then you can find the full reference in the alphabetized list that follows.

Introduction

- When God gives a gift: Card (2000).

Introducing the Home Security System and the Lipid Neighborhood

- Lp(a) 6.5x as atherogenic: Bjornson et al (2024).
- Coronary artery calcium scan radiation dose: Allio et al (2022).

Home Security System Pillar 1: Normalize Blood Sugar

- Insulin and glucose physiology: Nelson and Cox (2013).
- Suitcase analogy: Attia and Fung (episode from 2019).
- Independent hyperinsulinemia and all-cause mortality: Acevedo-Fernandez (2023).
- Hyperinsulinemia and hyperglycemia mortality: Wang et al (2023).
- Insulin and eNOS: Muniyappa and Sowers (2013).
- Insulin, obesity and cancer: Pati et al (2023).
- 2-4x risk of CAD mortality in diabetes: Aronson and Edelman (2014).
- GLP-1 and M1 to M2 macrophage polarization: Chen et al (2022).
- Glucose in the brain: Cunnane et al (2020), Kyrtata et al (2021), de leon et al (1983), Gudala et al (2013), Raut et al (2023).
- Hyperglycemia and sorbitol dehydrogenase: Singh et al (2021).
- FGF21: Rose et al (2025).
- C-peptide: Leighton et al (2017), Patel et al (2012).
- Insulin 18-40 units under normal physiologic conditions: Ramchandani et al (2010).
- EGFR below 75 and all-cause mortality: Hallan et al (2012).
- Low Muscle Mass and CAC: Ko et al (2016).
- Sleep deprivation quickest way to insulin resistance: Knutson and Cauter (2015).
- Protein metaphor for fuel usage: Attia and Galpin (episode from 2023).
- Mitochondria and GLUT4: Nelson and Cox (2013).
- Review of Diabetes Medications: Weinberg Sibony et al (2023).
- Pioglitazone and HF: Clarke et al (2017).

- SGLT2i and epicardial fat reduction: Masson et al (2021).
- MTORC1, exercise, and leucine: D'Hulst et al (2022).

Home Security System Pillar 2: Keep Blood Pressure Normal

- BP Physiology: Costanzo (2018), Fuchs and Whelton (2020).
- Licorice and BP: Geijerstam et al (2024).
- Metabolic effects of fructose: Kutlu Inci et al (2022).
- Uric acid and CAC progression: Liang et al (2019).
- Systemic effects of alcohol: Varghese and Dakhode (2022), Nelson and Cox (2013), LeClair (no year).
- EPIC-NORFOLK study and increased risk of mortality with microalbuminuria: Yuyun et al (2004).

Home Security System Pillar 3: Keep Inflammation Low

- IL-6 and exercise: Docherty et al (2022).
- IL-6 genetics and CAD: Yao et al (2023), Ferreira et al (2024).
- Tsimane: Vasunilashorn et al (2010).
- CANTOS trial and inflammation: Aday and Riker (2018).
- CRP and GlycA: Akinkuolie et al (2016).
- CRP and waist circumference: Nakamura et al (2008).
- C5, MAC and plaque: Martinez-Lopez et al (2020).

Home Security System Pillar 4: Smoking and Drugs

If you need references here, other help is emergent and necessary.

Part 2: The Lipid Neighborhood

- Lipoprotein physiology, structure, and teleology: Feingold (2021), Nelson and Cox (2013).
- Every cell can synthesize its own cholesterol: Duan et al (2022)
- Size of particles <70 nm potentially entering arterial intima: Ginsberg et al (2021).
- Majority of atherogenic particles are LDL: Jang et al (2020).
- Superiority of ApoB as a particle metric: Ahmad et al (2023).
- Postprandial lipemia and remnant particles: Drexel et al (2024), Ginsberg et al (2021), Packard et al (2020)
- Triglyceride-rich remnants 4x as atherogenic: Bjornson et al (2024).
- Small dense LDL: Ikezaki et al (2021), Krauss (2022).
- ApoC3: Packard et al (2020).
- Major players in clearance: Cohen et al (2006), Seidah and Prat (2022), Endo (2010).
- GOLIATH: Clifford et al (2020).

HDL: The Good Cholesterol

- J Curve with mortality: Liu et al (2022).
- Complexity of HDL and failure of HDL-raising therapeutics: Woudberg et al (2018).
- Endogenous and Exogenous Pathways: Feingold (2021), Nelson and Cox (2013), Attia and Dayspring (episode from 2018).
- Reverse LPS transport: Dusuel et al (2020) and Levels et al (2005).
- Postprandial low HDL: Kolovou et al (2004).
- CETP and HDL: Nurmohamed et al (2022).

- Insulin resistance without high trigs in those of African descent: Sumner et al (2005).
- Serum amyloid A and dysfunctional HDL: Wilson et al (2018).
- Number of cholesterol particles on HDL and LDL: Hevonoja et al (2004).

Lp(a): The "Felon" of the Lipid Neighborhood

- 28% increased risk per 50 nmol/L: Bjornson et al (2024).
- History and association with CV events: Nordestgaard et al (2024), Kronenberg et al (2022).
- Lp(a) and preeclampsia: Galani et al (2025).
- Lp(a) and keloid: Ruder et al (2022).
- Genetics of Lp(a): Arsenault and Kamstrup (2022).
- Risk increasing above 30 mg/dL: Raitakari et al (2023).
- Inflammatory component of Lp(a): Dzobo et al (2022).
- Menopause and Lp(a): Corral et al (2024).
- Atherogenicity not due to ApoB: Trinder et al (2021).
- Statins and residual risk in those with Lp(a) >50 mg/dL: Willeit et al (2018).
- Statins increase Lp(a) 19.3%: Zhu et al (2022).
- Potential therapeutics for Lp(a): Youssef et al (2023), Nordestgaard et al (2024).

Understanding Your Cholesterol Panel

- Ratios involved in lipid panel calculations: Berberich and Hegele (2022).
- ApoB as a biomarker from CARDIA: Wilkins et al (2016).
- Discordance between mass and particles: Fuior and Gafencu (2019).

- Residual elevation in ApoB and non-HDL-c 82% increased risk: Johannesen et al (2025).
- LDL-Triglycerides: Clifford et al (2023).
- Insulin resistance starting in skeletal muscle: Song et al (2020).
- Desmosterol and Alzheimer's Disease: Sato et al (2012) and Sato et al (2015), Sittiwet et al (2018).
- APOE4 carriers being hyperabsorbers: Dayspring et al (2015).
- LP-IR in MESA and Women's Health Studies: Mackey et al (2015), Harada et al (2017).
- Increased VLDL-p size with low-carb diet: Westman et al (2006).
- Increased VLDL-p size with PCSK9 inhibition: Masuda et al (2020).
- HDL-p in clinical trials: Kontush (2015).
- Risk-Enhancing factors: Mach et al (2020).
- Erectile Dysfunction: Nannas et al (2021), Mei et al (2024).

Imaging: Identification of Disease

- ICONIC data showing 2/3 of MI in a non-stenotic vessel: Chang et al (2019).
- Utility of CAC: Budoff et al (2010), Cheong et al (2021).
- CAC score of 300 equivalent to secondary prevention: Budoff et al (2023).
- CAC in CARDIA in young people: Carr et al (2017).
- CAC in FH: Mimame et al (2019).
- Warranty of CAC: Valenti et al (2015).
- CAC of zero and NNT of 3571 to infinite: Mitchell et al (2018).
- 1 msv of radiation with CCTA: Richards and Obaid (2019).

- Mean age of incident CAC in white males 36: Yeboah-Kordieh et al (2025).
- PROMISE and Functional Testing: Hoffmann et al (2017).
- High-risk plaque features: Dawson and Layland (2022).
- Thoracic Arterial Calcification from MESA: Brodov et al (2015).
- CCTA and Miami Heart Study: Hagan et al (2024).
- Vulnerable plaque: Sakamoto et al (2022).
- PESA and carotid/iliofemoral ultrasound: Ibanez et al (2021).
- The Power of 1%: Bhindi et al (2019).
- REVERSAL, ASTEROID, and SATURN statin trials on plaque: Stegman et al (2016).
- Effect of statins and PCSK9 inhibition on coronary plaque: Marfella et al (2023), Nicholls et al (2016) and Nicholls et al (2022), Kataoka et al (2024), Raber et al (2022).
- High-intensity interval training and plaque regression: Vesterbekkmo et al (2023).

Guidelines and How Low is Too Low?

- Guidelines references: Mach et al (2020), Virani et al (2023).
- Copenhagen Baby Heart Study: Nielsen et al (2023).
- Low LDL-c, HDL and sepsis: De Geest and Mishra (2022).
- Long-term low LDL-c levels with PCSK9 inhibition: Zimmerman et al (2023), O'Donoghue et al (2022).
- 43% fewer CV events in those with low LDL-c on PCSK9 inhibitor: Gaba et al (2023).

The Tools in the Lipid-Lowering Toolbox

- Cholestyramine and Fibrates: Pedersen (2016).
- Statin history: Endo (2010)
- Statin pleiotropy: Liao and Laufs (2005).
- SAMSON trial showing nocebo effect in myalgias: Krishnamurthy et al (2022).
- Statins reduce muscle mitochondrial function >30% in asymptomatic people: Ryan et al (2024).
- Pro athletes and statins: Sinzinger and O'Grady (2004).
- Creatine for SAMS: Scarsi et al (2024).
- 10% vs 36% increase in diabetes with higher intensity statin: CTTC (2024).
- Statins and GGPP: Wang et al (2022), Macchi et al (2019).
- Statins reduce GLP-1: She et al (2024).
- Exercise in animals abrogates muscle mitochondrial dysfunction with statins: Seo et al (2020).
- Controversy on statins and dementia: Schultz et al (2018)
- Rule of 6% with statin doubling: Cai et al (2014).
- RACING trial of combo therapy with ezetimibe: Kim et al (2022).
- Ezetimibe and UDCA for gallstones: Lee et al (2024).
- Statins increase PCSK9 levels: Macchi et al (2019).
- Non-statin medication review: Bardolia et al (2021).
- EWTOPIA trial ezetimibe: Ouchi et al (2019).
- CLEAR outcomes bempedoic acid: Nissen et al (2023).
- 100% of PCSK9 inhibited within 4 hours: Leucker et al (2020).
- Review of PCSK9 inhibition FOURIER and ODYSSEY: Furtado and Giugliano (2020).
- ORION-3 study of inclisiran: Ray et al (2023).
- EPA mechanism of action: Sherratt et al (2020).

- Omega-3 Index: Harris et al (2017).
- CETP Inhibition History: Chang et al (2024).
- Supplements: Mirzai and Laffin (2023).
- Nattokinase and carotid plaque: Chen et al (2022).
- Citrus bergamot: Carpenito et al (2025) and Huang et al (2021).

The Endocrine Thermostat: Thyroid and Adrenal Function

- Endocrine disease and effect on lipids: Feingold (2023).
- HPT and HPA axes for thyroid and adrenal function: Costanzo (2018).
- Thyroid and lipids: Rizos et al (2011).
- Thyroid supplements: Desai and Bernet (2025).

The Dark Arts of Hormone Replacement Therapy

- Menopausal HRT: van Oortmerssen et al (2025), Waters et al (2002).
- KEEPS: Miller et al (2019).
- TRAVERSE trial: Lincoff et al (2023).
- Icelandic HRT: Gudmundsson et al (2016)
- Testosterone and effects on plaque and glycosaminoglycans: Kumarapperuma et al (2024), Gencer et al (2021).
- Preserving muscle mass while on ADT: Overkamp et al (2023).

Oxytocin

- Intranasal oxytocin: Espinoza et al (2021).

Prolactin, Growth Hormone, and Parathyroid Hormone

- Hyperprolactinemia and lipids/metabolism: Schwetz et al (2016), Pirchio et al (2022).
- PTH and atherosclerosis in athletes: Claessen et al (2025), Celeski et al (2024).

The Deep End of the Community Pool

Conditions of Low HDL and LDL Cholesterol

- Hypobetalipoproteinemia: Welty et al (1997).
- LCAT deficiency and Lipoprotein X: Ossoli et al (2016).
- MVX: Li et al (2025).
- Various Lipid disorders: Kalwick and Roth (2025).

Bile Acids

- Bile acid metabolism: Fleishman and Kumar (2024).

LPL and Chylomicronemia

- Chylomicronemia: Saadatagah et al (2025).
- FCS and MCT: Williams et al (2018).
- Non-hydrolytic function of LPL: Zheng et al (2011).
- Type III Dysbetalipoproteinemia: Berberich and Hegele (2022).

The ANGPTL Family

- ANGPTL Physiology: Chen et al (2023), Thorin et al (2023).

- Diabetes and DVT: Deischinger et al (2022).

The Intracellular Cholesterol Relay

- Cholesterol homeostasis: Feingold (2021), Nelson and Cox (2013).
- Vitamin D and cholesterol homeostasis: Songtao Li et al (2016).
- Saturated Fat: Perna and Hewlings (2022).
- Fiber: Di Rosa et al (2022).
- Imidazole propionate: Mastrangelo et al (2025).

Factors Beyond ApoB

- Transcytosis: Zhang and Fernandez-Hernando 2020, Bolanle et al (2025).
- Mucopolysaccharidosis and vascular disease Braunlin et al (2011).
- 9p21.3: Salido et al (2025).

Autophagy

- MTORC1, exercise, and leucine: D'Hulst et al (2022).
- Statins, FOXO1 and atrogin-1: Zhao et al (2025).

Lean Mass Hyper-Responders

- KETO-CTA: Soto-Mota et al (2025).
- Lipid energy model: Norwitz et al (2022).
- NATURE-CT: Aldana et al (2024).
- Free fatty acids primary source: Koutsari et al (2013).
- Insulin and bile acids: Cortes and Eckel (2022).
- Direct LDL secretion: Skogsberg et al (2008).

- FXR and ApoB production: Hanniman et al (2005).
- Insulin and cholesterol absorption: Hasebe et al (2022).
- Hepatocyte cholesterol handling and shunt pathways: Scott Kiss and Sniderman (2017).

Cholesterol in the Brain

- APOE4 risk of Alzheimer's: Yassine et al (2017).
- CAC and Dementia from MESA: Fujiyoshi et al (2017).
- ASCVD and 29% increased dementia incidence: Liang et al (2023).
- Exercise and dementia: Pahlavani (2023).
- High Cardiorespiratory fitness and decreased dementia: Anderer (2025).
- Hyperinsulinemia and dementia: Luchsinger et al (2004).
- Diabetes, obesity, and dementia: Gudala et al (2013) and Raji et al (2023).
- Niemann-Pick C Disease: Wheeler and Sillence (2020).
- APOE4 contribution to dementia: Loving and Bruce (2020), Khalil et al (2021), Krogsaeter et al (2023), Mahley (2016).
- Alzheimer's biomarkers, amyloid and tau: Angioni et al (2022), Niotis et al (2024), Varma et al (2021), Kent et al (2020).
- Oxysterols and impaired cholesterol elimination in the brain: Gamba et al (2021), Anderson et al (2020), Fitz et al (2019).
- Decreased cholesterol synthesis in the brain: Sato et al (2015), Bai et al (2022), Sittiwet et al (2018).
- PCSK9 in the brain elevated in ApoE4 carriers: Simeone et al (2021), Picard et al (2022).
- PCSK9 in the brain: Papotti et al (2022), Vilella et al (2024).

- BDNF and cholesterol in neurons: Spagnuolo et al (2018).

FAQ

- Creatine: Post et al (2019).
- Sauna: Laukkanen et al (2016).
- Cold and PGC1α: Liang and Ward (2006).
- Cardiorespiratory fitness and mortality: Kokkinos et al (2022).
- Coffee: van Tol et al (1997).
- Fatty streaks in human fetuses: Napoli et al (1997).

Appendix A:

- DNP Toxicity: Grundlingh et al (2011).
- Discovery of GLP-1RA: Eng et al (1992) and Raufman (1996).
- History of cholesterol: Kuijpers (2021).

REFERENCES

Aberra, T., Peterson, E.D., Pagidipati, N.J., Mulder, H., Wojdyla, D.M., Philip, S., Granowitz, C., Navar, A.M. (2020). The association between triglycerides and incident cardiovascular disease: what is "optimal?" *Journal of Clinical Lipidology*, 14, 438-447. doi:10.1016/j.jacl.2020.04.009.

Acevedo-Fernández, M., Porchia, L. M., Elguezabal-Rodelo, R. G., López-Bayghen, E., & Gonzalez-Mejia, M. E. (2023). Concurrence of hyperinsulinemia and hyperuricemia significantly augmented all-cause mortality. *Nutrition, Metabolism, and Cardiovascular Diseases: NMCD*, *33*(9), 1725–1732. doi.org/10.1016/j.numecd.2023.05.023

Aday, A. W., & Ridker, P. M. (2018). Anti-inflammatory therapy in clinical care: The CANTOS trial and beyond. *Frontiers in Cardiovascular Medicine*, *5*, 62. https://doi.org/10.3389/fcvm.2018.00062

Af Geijerstam, P., Joelsson, A., Rådholm, K., & Nyström, F. H. (2024). A low dose of daily licorice intake affects renin, aldosterone, and home blood pressure in a randomized crossover trial. *The American Journal of Clinical Nutrition*, *119*(3), 682–691. https://doi.org/10.1016/j.ajcnut.2024.01.011

Ahmad, M., Sniderman, A. D., & Hegele, R. A. (2023). Apolipoprotein B in cardiovascular risk assessment. *CMAJ : Canadian Medical Association Journal*, *195*(33), E1124. https://doi.org/10.1503/cmaj.230048

Akinkuolie, A. O., Glynn, R. J., Padmanabhan, L., Ridker, P. M., & Mora, S. (2016). Circulating N-linked glycoprotein side-chain biomarker, rosuvastatin therapy, and incident cardiovascular disease: An analysis from the JUPITER Trial. *Journal of the American Heart Association*, *5*(7), e003822. doi.org/10.1161/JAHA.116.003822

Allio, I. R., Caobelli, F., Popescu, C. E., Haaf, P., Alberts, I., Frey, S. M., & Zellweger, M. J. (2023). Low-dose coronary artery calcium scoring compared to the standard protocol. *Journal of Nuclear Cardiology: Official Publication of the American Society of Nuclear Cardiology*, *30*(3), 1191–1198. https://doi.org/10.1007/s12350-022-03120-3

Anderer S. (2025) Cardiorespiratory fitness in middle and older age is associated with lower dementia risk. *JAMA*, *333*(4):280. https://doi:10.1001/jama.2024.25517

Anderson, A., Campo, A., Fulton, E., Corwin, A., Jerome, W. G., 3rd, & O'Connor, M. S. (2020). 7-Ketocholesterol in disease and aging. *Redox Biology*, *29*, 101380. https://doi.org/10.1016/j.redox.2019.101380

Angioni, D., Delrieu, J., Hansson, O., Fillit, H., Aisen, P., Cummings, J., Sims, J.R., Braunstein, J.B., Sabbagh, M., Bittner, T., Pontecorvo, M., Bozeat, S., Dage, J.L., Largent, E., Mattke, S., Correa, O., Gutierrez Robledo, L.M.,

Baldivieso, V., Willis, D.R., Atri, A., Bateman, R.J., Ousset, P.J., Vellas, B., & Weiner, M. (2022). Blood biomarkers from research use to clinical practice: What must be done? A report from the EU/US CTAD Task Force. *Journal of Preventative Alzheimer's Disease, 9*(4), 569-579. doi: 10.14283/jpad.2022.85.

Arsenault, B. J., & Kamstrup, P. R. (2022). Lipoprotein(a) and cardiovascular and valvular diseases: A genetic epidemiological perspective. *Atherosclerosis*, *349*, 7–16. doi.org/10.1016/j.atherosclerosis.2022.04.015

Attia, P. (Host) & Dayspring, T. (Guest). Part II of V: Lipid metrics, lipid measurements, and cholesterol regulation. Available at https://peterattiamd.com/tomdayspring2/. Accessed May 2, 2024.

Attia, P. (Host) & Fung, J (Guest). Fasting as a potent antidote to obesity, insulin resistance, type 2 diabetes, and the many symptoms of metabolic illness. Available at peterattiamd.com/jasonfung/. Accessed August 3, 2024.

Attia, P. (Host), & Galpin A. (Guest). The science of strength, muscle, and training for longevity. Available at https://peterattiamd.com/andygalpin/. Accessed April 28, 2024.

Attiq, A., Afzal, S., Ahmad, W., & Kandeel, M. (2024). Hegemony of inflammation in atherosclerosis and coronary artery disease. *European Journal of Pharmacology*, 176338. doi.org/10.1016/j.ejphar.2024.176338.

Bai, X., Mai, M., Yao, K. *et al.* The role of DHCR24 in the pathogenesis of AD: re-cognition of the relationship between cholesterol and AD pathogenesis. *Acta Neuropathologica Communications, 10*, 35 (2022). doi.org/10.1186/s40478-022-01338-3.

Bao, X., Liang, Y., Chang, H., Cai, T., Feng, B., Gordon, K., Zhu, Y., Shi, H., He, Y., & Xie, L. (2024). Targeting proprotein convertase subtilisin/kexin type 9 (PCSK9): From bench to bedside. *Signal Transduction and Targeted Therapy*, *9*(1), 13. doi.org/10.1038/s41392-023-01690-3.

Bardolia, C., Nashita, S. A., & Turgeon, J. (2021). Emerging non-statin treatment options for lowering low-density lipoprotein cholesterol. *Frontiers in Cardiovascular Medicine, 17*(8). doi.org/10.3389/fcvm.2021.789931.

Basiak, M., Kosowski, M., Hachula, M., & Okopien, B. (2022). Impact of PCSK9 inhibition on proinflammatory cytokines and matrix metalloproteinases release in patients with mixed hyperlipidemia and vulnerable atherosclerotic plaque. *Pharmaceuticals (Basel, Switzerland)*, *15*(7), 802. doi.org/10.3390/ph15070802.

Benitez, S., Puig, N., Rives, J., Solé, A., & Sánchez-Quesada, J. L. (2023). Can electronegative LDL act as a multienzymatic complex? *International Journal of Molecular Sciences*, *24*(8), 7074. https://doi.org/10.3390/ijms24087074

Berberich, A. J., & Hegele, R. A. (2022). A modern approach to dyslipidemia. *Endocrine Reviews*, *43*(4), 611–653. doi.org/10.1210/endrev/bnab037

Bhindi, R., Guan, M., Zhao, Y., Humphries, K. H., & Mancini, G. B. J. (2019). Coronary atheroma regression and adverse cardiac events: A systematic review and meta-regression analysis. *Atherosclerosis*, *284*, 194–201. doi.org/10.1016/j.atherosclerosis.2019.03.005

Bi, Y., Li, M., Liu, Y., Li, T., Lu, J., Duan, P., Xu, F., Dong, Q., Wang, A., Wang, T., Zheng, R., Chen, Y., Xu, M., Wang, X., Zhang, X., Niu, Y., Kang, Z., Lu, C., Wang, J., Qiu, X., ... BPROAD Research Group (2024). Intensive blood pressure control in patients with type 2 diabetes. *The New England Journal of Medicine*, 10.1056/NEJMoa2412006. Advance online publication. https://doi.org/10.1056/NEJMoa2412006

Björnson, E., Adiels, M., Gummesson, A., Taskinen, M. R., Burgess, S., Packard, C. J., & Borén, J. (2024). Quantifying triglyceride-rich lipoprotein atherogenicity, associations with inflammation, and implications for risk assessment using non-HDL cholesterol. *Journal of the American College of Cardiology*, *84*(14), 1328–1338. https://doi.org/10.1016/j.jacc.2024.07.034

Björnson, E., Adiels, M., Taskinen, M. R., Burgess, S., Chapman, M. J., Packard, C. J., & Borén, J. (2024). Lipoprotein(a) is markedly more atherogenic than LDL: An apolipoprotein B-based genetic analysis. *Journal of the American College of Cardiology*, *83*(3), 385–395. https://doi.org/10.1016/j.jacc.2023.10.039

Borràs, C., Mercer, A., Sirisi, S., Alcolea, D., Escolà-Gil, J.C., Blanco-Vaca, F., & Tondo M. (2022). HDL-like-mediated cell cholesterol trafficking in the Central Nervous System and Alzheimer's disease pathogenesis. *International Journal of Molecular Sciences,* 23(16):9356. doi.org/10.3390/ijms23169356.

Budoff, M. J., Hokanson, J. E., Nasir, K., Shaw, L. J., Kinney, G. L., Chow D., Demoss, D., Nuguri, V., Nabavi, V., Ratakonda, R., Berman, D. S., & Raggi, P. (2010). Progression of coronary artery calcium predicts all-cause mortality. *JACC Cardiovascular Imaging*, *3*(12), 1229–1236. doi.org/10.1016/j.jcmg.2010.08.018

Budoff, M. J., Kinninger, A., Gransar, H., Achenbach, S., Al-Mallah, M., Bax, J. J., Berman, D. S., Cademartiri, F., Callister, T. Q., Chang, H. J., Chow, B. J. W., Cury, R. C., Feuchtner, G., Hadamitzky, M., Hausleiter, J., Kaufmann, P. A., Leipsic, J., Lin, F. Y., Kim, Y. J., Marques, H., ... CONFIRM Investigators (2023). When does a calcium score equate to secondary prevention?: Insights from the multinational CONFIRM registry. *JACC Cardiovascular imaging*, *16*(9), 1181–1189. doi.org/10.1016/j.jcmg.2023.03.008

Budoff, M. J., Kinninger, A., Gransar, H., Achenbach, S., Al-Mallah, M., Bax, J. J., Berman, D. S., Cademartiri, F., Callister, T. Q., Chang, H. J., Chow, B. J. W., Cury, R. C., Feuchtner, G., Hadamitzky, M., Hausleiter, J., Kaufmann, P. A., Leipsic, J., Lin, F. Y., Kim, Y. J., Marques, H., ... CONFIRM Investigators. (2023). When does a calcium score equate to secondary prevention? Insights from the multinational CONFIRM registry. *JACC Cardiovascular Imaging*, *16*(9), 1181–1189. doi.org/10.1016/j.jcmg.2023.03.008.

Cai, R., Yuan, Y., Zhou, Y., Xia, W., Wang, P., Sun, H., Yang, Y., Huang, R., & Wang, S. (2014). Lower intensified target LDL-c level of statin therapy results in a higher risk of incident diabetes: a meta-analysis. *PloS one*, *9*(8), e104922. https://doi.org/10.1371/journal.pone.0104922

Card, M. (2000). *The Walk*. Thomas Nelson, Inc.

Carpenito, M., Coletti, F., Muscoli, S., Guarino, L., Di Cristo, A., Cammalleri, V.,

Mega, S., Emerenziani, S., Cicala, M., Fanali, C., Ussia, G. P., & Grigioni, F. (2025). Unveiling the power of bergamot: Beyond lipid-lowering effects. *Nutrients, 17*(11), 1871. https://doi.org/10.3390/nu17111871

Carr, J. J., Jacobs, D. R., Jr, Terry, J. G., Shay, C. M., Sidney, S., Liu, K., Schreiner, P. J., Lewis, C. E., Shikany, J. M., Reis, J. P., & Goff, D. C., Jr (2017). Association of coronary artery calcium in adults aged 32 to 46 years with incident coronary heart disease and death. *JAMA Cardiology, 2*(4), 391–399. https://doi.org/10.1001/jamacardio.2016.5493

Carson, J. A. S., Lichtenstein, A. H., Anderson, C. A. M., Appel, L. J., Kris-Etherton, P. M., Meyer, K. A., Petersen, K., Polonsky, T., Van Horn, L., & American Heart Association Nutrition Committee of the Council on Lifestyle and Cardiometabolic Health; Council on Arteriosclerosis, Thrombosis and Vascular Biology; Council on Cardiovascular and Stroke Nursing; Council on Clinical Cardiology; Council on Peripheral Vascular Disease; and Stroke Council (2020). Dietary cholesterol and cardiovascular risk: A science advisory from the American Heart Association. *Circulation, 141*(3), e39–e53. https://doi.org/10.1161/CIR.0000000000000743

Chang, H. J., Lin, F. Y., Lee, S. E., Andreini, D., Bax, J., Cademartiri, F., Chinnaiyan, K., Chow, B. J. W., Conte, E., Cury, R. C., Feuchtner, G., Hadamitzky, M., Kim, Y. J., Leipsic, J., Maffei, E., Marques, H., Plank, F., Pontone, G., Raff, G. L., van Rosendael, A. R., ... Min, J. K. (2018). Coronary atherosclerotic precursors of acute coronary syndromes. *Journal of the American College of Cardiology, 71*(22), 2511–2522. https://doi.org/10.1016/j.jacc.2018.02.079

Chen, H., Chen, J., Zhang, F., Li, Y., Wang, R., Zheng, Q., Zhang, X., Zeng, J., Xu, F., & Lin, Y. (2022). Effective management of atherosclerosis progress and hyperlipidemia with nattokinase: A clinical study with 1,062 participants. *Frontiers in Cardiovascular Medicine, 9*, 964977. https://doi.org/10.3389/fcvm.2022.964977

Chen, J., Mei, A., Wei, Y., Li, C., Qian, H., Min, X., Yang, H., Dong, L., Rao, X., & Zhong, J. (2022). GLP-1 receptor agonist as a modulator of innate immunity. *Frontiers in Immunology, 13*, 997578. https://doi.org/10.3389/fimmu.2022.997578

Chen, Z., Shao, W., Li, Y., Zhang, X., Geng, Y., Ma, X., Tao, B., Ma, Y., Yi, C., Zhang, B., Zhang, R., Lin, J., & Chen, J. (2024). Inhibition of PCSK9 prevents and alleviates cholesterol gallstones through PPARα-mediated CYP7A1 activation. *Metabolism: Clinical and Experimental, 152*, 155774. doi.org/10.1016/j.metabol.2023.155774

Cheong, B. Y. C., Wilson, J. M., Spann, S. J., Pettigrew, R. I., Preventza, O. A., & Muthupillai, R. (2021). Coronary artery calcium scoring: An evidence-based guide for primary care physicians. *Journal of Internal Medicine, 289*(3), 309–324. doi.org/10.1111/joim.13176

Cholesterol Treatment Trialists' (CTT) Collaboration. (2024). Effects of statin therapy on diagnoses of new-onset diabetes and worsening glycaemia in large-scale randomized blinded statin trials: An individual participant data meta-analysis. *The Lancet. Diabetes & Endocrinology, 12*(5), 306–319. doi.org/10.1016/S2213-8587(24)00040-8

Cibičková L. (2011). Statins and their influence on brain cholesterol. *Journal of Clinical Lipidology*, *5*(5), 373–379. https://doi.org/10.1016/j.jacl.2011.06.007

Climent, E., Benaiges, D., & Pedro-Botet, J. (2021). Hydrophilic or lipophilic statins?. *Frontiers in Cardiovascular Medicine, 8*, 687585. https://doi.org/10.3389/fcvm.2021.687585

Cohen, J. C., Boerwinkle, E., Mosley, T. H., Jr, & Hobbs, H. H. (2006). Sequence variations in PCSK9, low LDL, and protection against coronary heart disease. *The New England Journal of Medicine, 354*(12), 1264–1272. doi.org/10.1056/NEJMoa054013.

Corral, P., Matta, M.G., Aguilar-Salinas, C., Mehta, R., Berg, G., Ruscica, M., & Schreier, L. (2024) Lipoprotein(a) throughout life in women, *American Journal of Preventive Cardiology, 20*(100885). doi.org/10.1016/j.ajpc.2024.100885.

Costanzo, L.S. (2018). *Physiology* (6th ed.). Elsevier Inc.

Cunnane S.C., Trushina, E., Morland, C., Prigione, A., Casadesus, G., Andrews, Z.B., Beal, M.F., Bergersen, L.H., Brinton, R.D., de la Monte, S., Eckert, A., Harvey, J., Jeggo, R., Jhamandas, J.H., Kann, O., la Cour, C.M., Martin, W.F., Mithieux, G., Moreira, P.I., Murphy, M.P., Nave, K.A., Nuriel, T., Oliet, S.H.R., Saudou, F., Mattson, M.P., Swerdlow, R.H., & Millan, M.J. (2020). Brain energy rescue: an emerging therapeutic concept for neurodegenerative disorders of ageing. *Nature Reviews Drug Discovery, 19*(9), 609-633. doi: 10.1038/s41573-020-0072-x.

Das Pradhan, A., Glynn, R. J., Fruchart, J. C., MacFadyen, J. G., Zaharris, E. S., Everett, B. M., Campbell, S. E., Oshima, R., Amarenco, P., Blom, D. J., Brinton, E. A., Eckel, R. H., Elam, M. B., Felicio, J. S., Ginsberg, H. N., Goudev, A., Ishibashi, S., Joseph, J., Kodama, T., Koenig, W., ... PROMINENT Investigators (2022). Triglyceride lowering with pemafibrate to reduce cardiovascular risk. *The New England journal of Medicine, 387*(21), 1923–1934. https://doi.org/10.1056/NEJMoa2210645

Dawson, L. P., Lum, M., Nerleker, N., Nicholls, S. J., & Layland, J. (2022). Coronary atherosclerotic plaque regression: JACC State-of-the-Art Review. *Journal of the American College of Cardiology, 79*(1), 66–82. https://doi.org/10.1016/j.jacc.2021.10.035

Dayspring, T. D., Varvel, S. A., Ghaedi, L., Thiselton, D. L., Bruton, J., & McConnell, J. P. (2015). Biomarkers of cholesterol homeostasis in a clinical laboratory database sample comprising 667,718 patients. Journal of Clinical Lipidology, 9(6), 807–816. doi.org/10.1016/j.jacl.2015.08.003.

De Geest, B., & Mishra, M. (2022). Impact of high-density lipoproteins on sepsis. *International Journal of Molecular Sciences, 23*(21), 12965. doi.org/10.3390/ijms232112965

de Leon, M. J., Ferris, S. H., George, A. E., Christman, D. R., Fowler, J. S., Gentes, C., Reisberg, B., Gee, B., Emmerich, M., Yonekura, Y., Brodie, J.,

Kricheff, I. I., & Wolf, A. P. (1983). Positron emission tomographic studies of aging and Alzheimer disease. *American Journal of Neuroradiology*, *4*(3), 568–571.

De Oliveira-Gomes, D., Joshi, P. H., Peterson, E. D., Rohatgi, A., Khera, A., & Navar, A. M. (2024). Apolipoprotein B: Bridging the gap between evidence and clinical practice. *Circulation*, *150*(1), 62–79. https://doi.org/10.1161/CIRCULATIONAHA.124.068885

D'Hulst, G., Masschelein, E., & De Bock, K. (2022). Resistance exercise enhances long-term mTORC1 sensitivity to leucine. *Molecular Metabolism*, *66*, 101615. https://doi.org/10.1016/j.molmet.2022.101615

Di Rosa, C., Altomare, A., Imperia, E., Spiezia, C., Khazrai, Y. M., & Guarino, M. P. L. (2022). The role of dietary fibers in the management of IBD symptoms. Nutrients, 14(22), 4775. https://doi.org/10.3390/nu14224777.

Docherty, S., Harley, R., McAuley, J. J., Crowe, L. A. N., Pedret, C., Kirwan, P. D., Siebert, S., & Millar, N. L. (2022). The effect of exercise on cytokines: Implications for musculoskeletal health: A narrative review. *BMC Sports Science, Medicine & Rehabilitation*, *14*(1), 5. https://doi.org/10.1186/s13102-022-00397-2

Drexel, H., Mader, A., Larcher, B., Festa, A., Vonbank, A., Fraunberger, P., Leiherer, A., & Saley, C. (2024). Remnent cholesterol and long-term incidence of death in coronary artery disease patients. *Atherosclerosis, 119048. https://www.atherosclerosis-journal.com/article/S0021-9150(24)01220-6/fulltext*

Duan, Y., Gong, K., Xu, S., Zhang, F., Meng, X., & Han, J. (2022). Regulation of cholesterol homeostasis in health and diseases: from mechanisms to targeted therapeutics. *Signal Transduction and Targeted Therapy*, *7*(1), 265. https://doi.org/10.1038/s41392-022-01125-5

Dusuel, A., Deckert, V., Pais de Barros, J. P., van Dongen, K., Choubley, H., Charron, É., Le Guern, N., Labbé, J., Mandard, S., Grober, J., Lagrost, L., & Gautier, T. (2021). Human cholesteryl ester transfer protein lacks lipopolysaccharide transfer activity, but worsens inflammation and sepsis outcomes in mice. *Journal of Lipid Research*, *62*, 100011. https://doi.org/10.1194/jlr.RA120000704

Dzobo, K. E., Kraaijenhof, J. M., Stroes, E. S. G., Nurmohamed, N. S., & Kroon, J. (2022). Lipoprotein(a): An underestimated inflammatory mastermind. *Atherosclerosis*, *349*, 101–109. doi.org/10.1016/j.atherosclerosis.2022.04.004

Endo A. (2010). A historical perspective on the discovery of statins. *Proceedings of the Japan Academy. Series B, Physical and biological sciences*, *86*(5), 484–493. doi.org/10.2183/pjab.86.484.

Eng, J., Kleinman, W. A., Singh, L., Singh, G., & Raufman, J. P. (1992). Isolation and characterization of exendin-4, an exendin-3 analogue, from Heloderma suspectum venom. Further evidence for an exendin receptor on dispersed acini from guinea pig pancreas. *The Journal of Biological Chemistry*, *267*(11), 7402–7405.

Enkhmaa, B., & Berglund, L. (2022). Non-genetic influences on lipoprotein(a) concentrations. *Atherosclerosis*, *349*, 53–62. https://doi.org/10.1016/j.atherosclerosis.2022.04.006

Feingold, K. R. (2024). Introduction to Lipids and Lipoproteins. In K.R. Feingold (Eds.) et. al., *Endotext*. MDText.com, Inc.

Ferreira, J.P., Vasques-Novoa, F., Neves, J.S., Zannad, F., & Leite-Moreira, A. (2024). Comparison of interleukin-6 and high-sensitivity C-reactive protein for cardiovascular risk assessment: Findings from the MESA study. *Atherosclerosis*, 117461. doi.org/10.1016/j.atherosclerosis.2024.117461.

Fitz, N. F., Nam, K. N., Koldamova, R., & Lefterov, I. (2019). Therapeutic targeting of nuclear receptors, liver X and retinoid X receptors, for Alzheimer's disease. *British Journal of Pharmacology*, *176*(18), 3599–3610. doi.org/10.1111/bph.14668.

Fuchs, F. D., & Whelton, P. K. (2020). High blood pressure and cardiovascular disease. *Hypertension Dallas, Texas: 1979*, *75*(2), 285–292. doi.org/10.1161/HYPERTENSIONAHA.119.14240

Fuior, E. V., & Gafencu, A. V. (2019). Apolipoprotein C1: Its pleiotropic effects in lipid metabolism and beyond. *International Journal of Molecular Sciences*, *20*(23), 5939. doi.org/10.3390/ijms20235939.

Fujiyoshi, A., Jacobs, D. R., Jr, Fitzpatrick, A. L., Alonso, A., Duprez, D. A., Sharrett, A. R., Seeman, T., Blaha, M. J., Luchsinger, J. A., & Rapp, S. R. (2017). Coronary artery calcium and risk of dementia in MESA (Multi-Ethnic Study of Atherosclerosis). *Circulation. Cardiovascular Imaging*, *10*(5), e005349. https://doi.org/10.1161/CIRCIMAGING.116.005349

Furtado, R. H. M., & Giugliano, R. P. (2020). What lessons have we learned and what remains to be clarified for PCSK9 Inhibitors? A review of FOURIER and ODYSSEY outcomes trials. *Cardiology and Therapy*, *9*(1), 59–73. doi.org/10.1007/s40119-020-00163-w.

Gaba, P., O'Donoghue, M. L., Park, J. G., Wiviott, S. D., Atar, D., Kuder, J. F., Im, K., Murphy, S. A., De Ferrari, G. M., Gaciong, Z. A., Toth, K., Gouni-Berthold, I., Lopez-Miranda, J., Schiele, F., Mach, F., Flores-Arredondo, J. H., López, J. A. G., Elliott-Davey, M., Wang, B., Monsalvo, M. L., ... Sabatine, M. S. (2023) Association between achieved low-density lipoprotein cholesterol levels and long-term cardiovascular and safety outcomes: An analysis of FOURIER-OLE. *Circulation*, *147*(16), 1192–1203. doi.org/10.1161/CIRCULATIONAHA.122.063399.

Galani, A., Zikopoulos, A., Potiris, A., Moustakli, E., Maneta-Stavrakaki, S., Paraskevaidi, M., Skentou, C., Zikopoulos, K., Drakakis, P., & Stavros, S. (2025). Exploring the impact of first trimester elevated lipoprotein(a) levels on preeclampsia, preterm delivery, and fetal growth restriction. *Journal of Clinical Medicine*, *14*(12), 4134. https://doi.org/10.3390/jcm14124134

Gamba, P., Giannelli, S., Staurenghi, E., Testa, G., Sottero, B., Biasi, F., Poli, G., & Leonarduzzi, G. (2021). The controversial role of 24-S-hydroxycholesterol in Alzheimer's disease. *Antioxidants (Basel, Switzerland)*, *10*(5), 740. doi.org/10.3390/antiox10050740.

Gao, Y., Shah, L. M., Ding, J., & Martin, S. S. (2023). US trends in cholesterol screening, lipid levels, and lipid-lowering medication use in US adults, 1999 to 2018. *Journal of the American Heart Association, 12*(3), e028205. https://doi.org/10.1161/JAHA.122.028205

Ginsberg, H. N., Packard, C. J., Chapman, M. J., Borén, J., Aguilar-Salinas, C. A., Averna, M., Ference, B. A., Gaudet, D., Hegele, R. A., Kersten, S., Lewis, G. F., Lichtenstein, A. H., Moulin, P., Nordestgaard, B. G., Remaley, A. T., Staels, B., Stroes, E. S. G., Taskinen, M. R., Tokgözoğlu, L. S., Tybjaerg-Hansen, A., ... Catapano, A. L. (2021). Triglyceride-rich lipoproteins and their remnants: Metabolic insights, role in atherosclerotic cardiovascular disease, and emerging therapeutic strategies. A consensus statement from the European Atherosclerosis Society. *European Heart Journal, 42*(47), 4791–4806. doi.org/10.1093/eurheartj/ehab551.

Glavinovic, T., Thanassoulis, G., de Graaf, J., Couture, P., Hegele, R. A., & Sniderman, A. D. (2022). Physiological bases for the superiority of apolipoprotein b over low-density lipoprotein cholesterol and non-high-density lipoprotein cholesterol as a marker of cardiovascular risk. *Journal of the American Heart Association, 11*(20). doi.org/10.1161/JAHA.122.025858

Grundlingh, J., Dargan, P. I., El-Zanfaly, M., & Wood, D. M. (2011). 2,4-dinitrophenol (DNP): A weight loss agent with significant acute toxicity and risk of death. *Journal of Medical Toxicology: Official Journal of the American College of Medical Toxicology*, 7(3), 205–212. https://doi.org/10.1007/s13181-011-0162-6

Gudala, K., Bansal, D., Schifano, F., & Bhansali, A. (2013). Diabetes mellitus and risk of dementia: A meta-analysis of prospective observational studies. *Journal of Diabetes Investigation*, 4(6), 640–650. doi.org/10.1111/jdi.12087.

Hagan, K., Mszar, R., Cainzos-Achirica, M., Blaha, M. J., Shapiro, M. D., Arias, L., Saxena, A., Cury, R., Budoff, M. J., Feldman, T., Fialkow, J., Al-Kindi, S., & Nasir, K. (2024). Low-density lipoprotein-cholesterol and subclinical coronary atherosclerosis in a middle-aged asymptomatic U.S. population: The Miami Heart Study at Baptist Health South Florida. *Atherosclerosis, 397*, 118551. doi.org/10.1016/j.atherosclerosis.2024.118551

Hallan, S.I., Matsushita, K., Sang, Y., et al. (2012). Age and association of kidney measures with mortality and end-stage renal disease. *JAMA, 308*(22): 2349–2360. doi:10.1001/jama.2012.16817

Hanniman, E. A., Lambert, G., McCarthy, T. C., & Sinal, C. J. (2005). Loss of functional farnesoid X receptor increases atherosclerotic lesions in apolipoprotein E-deficient mice. Journal of Lipid Research, 46(12), 2595–2604. https://doi.org/10.1194/jlr.M500390-JLR200

Hasebe, M., Iwasaki, Y., Keidai, Y., Iwasaki, K., Honjo, S., & Hamasaki, A. (2022). Plant sterol hyperabsorption caused by uncontrolled diabetes in a patient with a heterozygous ABCG5 variant. Journal of Diabetes Investigation, 13(11), 1934–1938. https://doi.org/10.1111/jdi.13874

Hevonoja, T., Pentikäinen, M. O., Hyvönen, M. T., Kovanen, P. T., & Ala-Korpela, M. (2000). Structure of low-density lipoprotein (LDL) particles:

Basis for understanding molecular changes in modified LDL. *Biochimica et biophysica acta*, *1488*(3), 189–210. doi.org/10.1016/s1388-1981(00)00123-2

Huang, Y., Tocmo, R., Nauman, M. C., Haughan, M. A., & Johnson, J. J. (2021). Defining the cholesterol lowering mechanism of bergamot (*Citrus bergamia*) extract in HepG2 and Caco-2 cells. *Nutrients*, *13*(9), 3156. https://doi.org/10.3390/nu13093156

Ibanez, B., Fernández-Ortiz, A., & Fernández-Friera, L. et al. (2021). Progression of early subclinical atherosclerosis (PESA) study: *JACC, 78*(2), 156–179 doi.org/10.1016/j.jacc.2021.05.011

Ikezaki, H., Lim, E., Cupples, L. A., Liu, C. T., Asztalos, B. F., & Schaefer, E. J. (2021). Small dense low-density lipoprotein cholesterol is the most atherogenic lipoprotein parameter in the prospective Framingham offspring study. *Journal of the American Heart Association*, *10*(5). doi.org/10.1161/JAHA.120.019140

Jang, E., Robert, J., Rohrer, L., von Eckardstein, A., & Lee, W. L. (2020). Transendothelial transport of lipoproteins. *Atherosclerosis*, *315*, 111–125. doi.org/10.1016/j.atherosclerosis.2020.09.020.

Kataoka, T., Morishita, T., Uzui, H., Sato, Y., Shimizu, T., Miyoshi, M., Yamaguchi, J., Shiomi, Y., Ikeda, H., Tama, N., Hasegawa, K., Ishida, K., & Tada, H. (2024). Very short-term effects of a single dose of a proprotein convertase subtilisin/kexin 9 inhibitor before percutaneous coronary intervention: A single-arm study. *Atherosclerosis*, 118581. doi.org/10.1016/j.atherosclerosis.2024.118581

Kent, S.A., Spires-Jones, T.L., & Durrant, C.S. (2020). The physiological roles of tau and Aβ: implications for Alzheimer's disease pathology and therapeutics. *Acta Neuropathologica, 140*(4), 417-447. doi: 10.1007/s00401-020-02196-w.

Khalil, Y. A., Rabès, J. P., Boileau, C., & Varret, M. (2021). APOE gene variants in primary dyslipidemia. *Atherosclerosis*, *328*, 11–22. doi.org/10.1016/j.atherosclerosis.2021.05.007.

Kim, B. K., Hong, S. J., Lee, Y. J., Hong, S. J., Yun, K. H., Hong, B. K., Heo, J. H., Rha, S. W., Cho, Y. H., Lee, S. J., Ahn, C. M., Kim, J. S., Ko, Y. G., Choi, D., Jang, Y., Hong, M. K., & RACING investigators (2022). Long-term efficacy and safety of moderate-intensity statin with ezetimibe combination therapy versus high-intensity statin monotherapy in patients with atherosclerotic cardiovascular disease (RACING): a randomized, open-label, non-inferiority trial. *Lancet (London, England)*, *400*(10349), 380–390. https://doi.org/10.1016/S0140-6736(22)00916-3

Knutson, K. L., & Van Cauter, E. (2008). Associations between sleep loss and increased risk of obesity and diabetes. *Annals of the New York Academy of Sciences*, *1129*, 287–304. https://doi.org/10.1196/annals.1417.033

Kolovou, G. D., Anagnostopoulou, K. K., Pilatis, N., Kafaltis, N., Sorodila, K., Psarros, E., & Cokkinos, D. V. (2004). Low fasting low high-density lipoprotein and postprandial lipemia. *Lipids in Health and Disease*, *3*, 18. doi.org/10.1186/1476-511X-3-18

Krauss R. M. (2022). Small dense low-density lipoprotein particles: Clinically relevant? *Current Opinion in Lipidology*, *33*(3), 160–166. doi.org/10.1097/MOL.0000000000000824

Krishnamurthy, A., Bradley, C., Ascunce, R., & Kim, S. M. (2022). SAMSON and the Nocebo Effect: Management of statin intolerance. *Current Cardiology Reports*, *24*(9), 1101–1108. doi.org/10.1007/s11886-022-01729-x.

Krogsaeter, E. K., McKetney, J., Marquez, A., Cakir, Z., Stevenson, E., Jang, G. M., Rao, A., Zhou, A., Huang, Y., Krogan, N. J., & Swaney, D. L. (2023). Lysosomal proteomics reveals mechanisms of neuronal apoE4-associated lysosomal dysfunction. *BioRxiv: The Preprint Server for Biology*, 2023.10.02.560519. doi.org/10.1101/2023.10.02.560519.

Kronenberg, F., Mora, S., Stroes, E. S. G., Ference, B. A., Arsenault, B. J., Berglund, L., Dweck, M. R., Koschinsky, M., Lambert, G., Mach, F., McNeal, C. J., Moriarty, P. M., Natarajan, P., Nordestgaard, B. G., Parhofer, K. G., Virani, S. S., von Eckardstein, A., Watts, G. F., Stock, J. K., Ray, K. K., ... Catapano, A. L. (2022). Lipoprotein(a) in atherosclerotic cardiovascular disease and aortic stenosis: A European Atherosclerosis Society consensus statement. *European Heart Journal*, *43*(39), 3925–3946. doi.org/10.1093/eurheartj/ehac361

Kronenberg, F., Mora, S., Stroes, E.S.G., Ference, B.A., Arsenault, B.J., Berglund, L., Dweck, M.R., Koschinsky, M., Lambert, G., Mach, F., McNeal, C.J., Moriarty, P.M., Natarajan, P., Nordestgaard, B.G., Parhofer, K.G., Virani, S.S., von Eckardstein, A., Watts, G.F., Stock, J.K., Ray, K.K., Tokgözoğlu, L.S., & Catapano, A.L. (2022). Lipoprotein(a) in atherosclerotic cardiovascular disease and aortic stenosis: A European Atherosclerosis Society consensus statement. *European Heart Journal, 43*(39), 3925-3946. doi: 10.1093/eurheartj/ehac361.

Kuijpers, P. M. J. C. (2021). History in medicine: The story of cholesterol, lipids and cardiology. *European Society of Cardiology, 19*(9), https://www.escardio.org/Journals/E-Journal-of-Cardiology-Practice/Volume-19/history-in-medicine-the-story-of-cholesterol-lipids-and-cardiology

Kyrtata, N., Emsley, H. C. A., Sparasci, O., Parkes, L. M., & Dickie, B. R. (2021). A systematic review of glucose transport alterations in Alzheimer's disease. *Frontiers in Neuroscience*, *15*, 626636. doi.org/10.3389/fnins.2021.626636.

Laukkanen, T., Kunutsor, S., Kauhanen, J., & Laukkanen, J. A. (2017). Sauna bathing is inversely associated with dementia and Alzheimer's disease in middle-aged Finnish men. *Age and Ageing*, *46*(2), 245–249. https://doi.org/10.1093/ageing/afw212

Lazar, A. N., Hanbouch, L., Boussicaut, L., Fourmaux, B., Daira, P., Millan, M. J., Bernoud-Hubac, N., & Potier, M. C. (2022). Lipid dys-homeostasis contributes to APOE4-associated AD pathology. *Cells*, *11*(22), 3616. doi.org/10.3390/cells11223616.

LeClair, R.J. (No year). Alcohol metabolism. *LibreText Medicine*. https://med.libretexts.org/Bookshelves/Basic_Science/Cell_Biology_Genetics_and_Biochemistry_for_Pre-Clinical_Students/09%

3A_Disorders_of_monosaccharide_metabolism_and_other_metabolic_conditions/9.02%3A_Alcohol_metabolism

Leighton, E., Sainsbury, C. A., & Jones, G. C. (2017). A practical review of c-peptide testing in diabetes. *Diabetes Therapy: Research, Treatment and Education of Diabetes and Related Disorders*, *8*(3), 475–487. https://doi.org/10.1007/s13300-017-0265-4

Leucker, T. M., Blaha, M. J., Jones, S. R., Vavuranakis, M. A., Williams, M. S., Lai, H., Schindler, T. H., Latina, J., Schulman, S. P., & Gerstenblith, G. (2020). Effect of evolocumab on atherogenic lipoproteins during the peri- and early postinfarction period: A placebo-controlled, randomized trial. *Circulation*, *142*(4), 419–421. https://doi.org/10.1161/CIRCULATIONAHA.120.046320

Levels, J. H., Marquart, J. A., Abraham, P. R., van den Ende, A. E., Molhuizen, H. O., van Deventer, S. J., & Meijers, J. C. (2005). Lipopolysaccharide is transferred from high-density to low-density lipoproteins by lipopolysaccharide-binding protein and phospholipid transfer protein. *Infection and Immunity*, *73*(4), 2321–2326. https://doi.org/10.1128/IAI.73.4.2321-2326.2005

Lexell J. (1995). Human aging, muscle mass, and fiber type composition. *The Journals of Gerontology. Series A, Biological Sciences and Medical ciences*, *50 Spec No*, 11–16. https://doi.org/10.1093/gerona/50a.special_issue.11

Liang, H., & Ward, W. F. (2006). PGC-1alpha: A key regulator of energy metabolism. *Advances in Physiology Education*, *30*(4), 145–151. https://doi.org/10.1152/advan.00052.2006

Liang, J., Li, C., Gao, D., Ma, Q., Wang, Y., Pan, Y., Zhang, W., Xie, W., & Zheng, F. (2023). Association between onset age of coronary heart disease and incident dementia: A prospective cohort study. *Journal of the American Heart Association*, *12*(23), e031407. doi.org/10.1161/JAHA.123.031407.

Liang, L., Hou, X., Bainey, K. R., Zhang, Y., Tymchak, W., Qi, Z., Li, W., & Banh, H. L. (2019). The association between hyperuricemia and coronary artery calcification development: A systematic review and meta-analysis. *Clinical Cardiology*, *42*(11), 1079–1086. https://doi.org/10.1002/clc.23266

Liao, J. K., & Laufs, U. (2005). Pleiotropic effects of statins. *Annual Review of Pharmacology and Toxicology*, *45*, 89–118. doi.org/10.1146/annurev.pharmtox.45.120403.095748

Liu, C., Dhindsa, D., Almuwaqqat, Z., Ko, Y. A., Mehta, A., Alkhoder, A. A., Alras, Z., Desai, S. R., Patel, K. J., Hooda, A., Wehbe, M., Sperling, L. S., Sun, Y. V., & Quyyumi, A. A. (2022). Association between high-density lipoprotein cholesterol levels and adverse cardiovascular outcomes in high-risk populations. *JAMA Cardiology*, *7*(7), 672–680. doi.org/10.1001/jamacardio.2022.0912.

Loving, B. A., & Bruce, K. D. (2020). Lipid and lipoprotein metabolism in microglia. *Frontiers in Physiology*, *11*, 393. doi.org/10.3389/fphys.2020.00393.

Loving, B. A., Tang, M., Neal, M. C., Gorkhali, S., Murphy, R., Eckel, R. H., & Bruce, K. D. (2021). Lipoprotein lipase regulates microglial lipid droplet accumulation. *Cells*, *10*(2), 198. doi.org/10.3390/cells10020198.

Luchsinger, J. A., Tang, M. X., Shea, S., & Mayeux, R. (2004). Hyperinsulinemia and risk of Alzheimer disease. *Neurology*, *63*(7), 1187–1192. https://doi.org/10.1212/01.wnl.0000140292.04932.87

Macchi, C., Ferri, N., Sirtori, C. R., Corsini, A., Banach, M., & Ruscica, M. (2021). Proprotein convertase subtilisin/kexin type 9: A view beyond the canonical cholesterol-lowering impact. *The American Journal of Pathology*, *191*(8), 1385–1397. https://doi.org/10.1016/j.ajpath.2021.04.016.

Mach, F., Baigent, C., Catapano, A. L., Koskinas, K. C., Casula, M., Badimon, L., Chapman, M. J., De Backer, G. G., Delgado, V., Ference, B. A., Graham, I. M., Halliday, A., Landmesser, U., Mihaylova, B., Pedersen, T. R., Riccardi, G., Richter, D. J., Sabatine, M. S., Taskinen, M. R., Tokgozoglu, L., ... ESC Scientific Document Group (2020). 2019 ESC/EAS Guidelines for the management of dyslipidaemias: Lipid modification to reduce cardiovascular risk. *European heart journal*, *41*(1), 111–188. https://doi.org/10.1093/eurheartj/ehz455

Mahley R. W. (2016). Central nervous system lipoproteins: ApoE and regulation of cholesterol metabolism. *Arteriosclerosis, Thrombosis, and Vascular Biology*, *36*(7), 1305–1315. doi.org/10.1161/ATVBAHA.116.307023.

Marfella, R., Prattichizzo, F., Sardu, C., Paolisso, P., D'Onofrio, N., Scisciola, L., La Grotta, R., Frigé, C., Ferraraccio, F., Panarese, I., Fanelli, M., Modugno, P., Calafiore, A.M., Melchionna, M., Sasso, F.C., Furbatto, F., D'Andrea, D., Siniscalchi, M., Mauro, C., Cesaro, A., Calabrò, P., Santulli, G., Balestrieri, M.L., Barbato, E., Ceriello, A., & Paolisso, G. (2023). Evidence of anti-inflammatory effect of PCSK9 inhibitors within the human atherosclerotic plaque, *Atherosclerosis, 16,* 1000-1006. doi.org/10.1016/j.atherosclerosis.2023.06.971.

Mendieta, G., Pocock, S., Mass, V., Moreno, A., Owen, R., García-Lunar, I., López-Melgar, B., Fuster, J. J., Andres, V., Pérez-Herreras, C., Bueno, H., Fernández-Ortiz, A., Sanchez-Gonzalez, J., García-Alvarez, A., Ibáñez, B., & Fuster, V. (2023). Determinants of progression and regression of subclinical atherosclerosis over 6 years. *Journal of the American College of Cardiology*, *82*(22), 2069–2083. https://doi.org/10.1016/j.jacc.2023.09.814

Miname, M. H., Bittencourt, M. S., Moraes, S. R., Alves, R. I. M., Silva, P. R. S., Jannes, C. E., Pereira, A. C., Krieger, J. E., Nasir, K., & Santos, R. D. (2019). Coronary artery calcium and cardiovascular events in patients with familial hypercholesterolemia receiving standard lipid-lowering therapy. *JACC. Cardiovascular Imaging*, *12*(9), 1797–1804. https://doi.org/10.1016/j.jcmg.2018.09.019

Mirzai, S., & Laffin, L. J. (2023). Supplements for lipid lowering: What does the evidence show? *Current Cardiology Reports*, *25*(8), 795–805. https://doi.org/10.1007/s11886-023-01903-9

Mitchell, J. D., Fergestrom, N., Gage, B. F., Paisley, R., Moon, P., Novak, E., Cheezum, M., Shaw, L. J., & Villines, T. C. (2018). Impact of statins on cardiovascular outcomes following coronary artery calcium scoring. *Journal of the*

American College of Cardiology, *72*(25), 3233–3242. doi.org/10.1016/j.jacc.2018.09.051

Monami, M., Sesti, G., & Mannucci, E. (2019). PCSK9 inhibitor therapy: A systematic review and meta-analysis of metabolic and cardiovascular outcomes in patients with diabetes. *Diabetes, Obesity & Metabolism*, *21*(4), 903–908. doi.org/10.1111/dom.13599.

Mora, S., Szklo, M., Otvos, J. D., Greenland, P., Psaty, B. M., Goff, D. C., Jr, O'Leary, D. H., Saad, M. F., Tsai, M. Y., & Sharrett, A. R. (2007). LDL particle subclasses, LDL particle size, and carotid atherosclerosis in the Multi-Ethnic Study of Atherosclerosis (MESA). *Atherosclerosis*, *192*(1), 211–217. https://doi.org/10.1016/j.atherosclerosis.2006.05.007

Muniyappa, R., & Sowers, J. R. (2013). Role of insulin resistance in endothelial dysfunction. *Reviews in Endocrine & Metabolic Disorders*, *14*(1), 5–12. doi.org/10.1007/s11154-012-9229-1

Nakamura, H., Ito, H., Egami, Y., Kaji, Y., Maruyama, T., Koike, G., Jingu, S., & Harada, M. (2008). Waist circumference is the main determinant of elevated C-reactive protein in metabolic syndrome. *Diabetes Research and Clinical Practice*, *79*(2), 330–336. https://doi.org/10.1016/j.diabres.2007.09.004

Neeland, I. J., Linge, J., & Birkenfeld, A. L. (2024). Changes in lean body mass with glucagon-like peptide-1-based therapies and mitigation strategies. *Diabetes, Obesity & Metabolism*, *26 Suppl 4*, 16–27. https://doi.org/10.1111/dom.15728

Nelson, D.L, & Cox, M.M. 2013. *Lehninger Principles of Biochemistry*. 6th ed. W.H. Freeman & Co.

Nicholls, S. J., Kataoka, Y., Nissen, S. E., Prati, F., Windecker, S., Puri, R., Hucko, T., Aradi, D., Herrman, J. R., Hermanides, R. S., Wang, B., Wang, H., Butters, J., Di Giovanni, G., Jones, S., Pompili, G., & Psaltis, P. J. (2022). Effect of evolocumab on coronary plaque phenotype and burden in statin-treated patients following myocardial infarction. *JACC. Cardiovascular Imaging*, *15*(7), 1308–1321. doi.org/10.1016/j.jcmg.2022.03.002.

Nicholls, S. J., Puri, R., Anderson, T., Ballantyne, C. M., Cho, L., Kastelein, J. J., Koenig, W., Somaratne, R., Kassahun, H., Yang, J., Wasserman, S. M., Scott, R., Ungi, I., Podolec, J., Ophuis, A. O., Cornel, J. H., Borgman, M., Brennan, D. M., & Nissen, S. E. (2016). Effect of evolocumab on progression of coronary disease in statin-treated patients: The GLAGOV Randomized Clinical Trial. *JAMA*, *316*(22), 2373–2384. doi.org/10.1001/jama.2016.16951.

Niotis, K., Saperia, C., & Saif, N. (2024). Alzheimer's disease risk reduction in clinical practice: A priority in the emerging field of preventive neurology. *National Mental Health*, *2*, 25–40. doi.org/10.1038/s44220-023-00191-0.

Nissen, S. E., Lincoff, A. M., Brennan, D., Ray, K. K., Mason, D., Kastelein, J. J. P., Thompson, P. D., Libby, P., Cho, L., Plutzky, J., Bays, H. E., Moriarty, P. M., Menon, V., Grobbee, D. E., Louie, M. J., Chen, C. F., Li, N., Bloedon, L., Robinson, P., Horner, M., ... CLEAR Outcomes Investigators (2023). Bempedoic acid and cardiovascular outcomes in statin-intolerant patients. *The New*

England Journal of Medicine, *388*(15), 1353–1364. https://doi.org/10.1056/NEJMoa2215024

No author. (2017). Diagram of major lipoprotein metabolism pathways. Lipids & Lipoproteins. https://basicmedicalkey.com/lipids-and-lipoproteins/#Bishop-ch015-fig003.

Nordestgaard B. G. (2017). A test in context: Lipid profile, fasting versus non-fasting. *Journal of the American College of Cardiology*, *70*(13), 1637–1646. https://doi.org/10.1016/j.jacc.2017.08.006

Nordestgaard, B. G., & Langsted, A. (2024). Lipoprotein(a) and cardiovascular disease. *Lancet (London, England)*, *404*(10459), 1255–1264. doi.org/10.1016/S0140-6736(24)01308-4

Nurmohamed, N. S., Ditmarsch, M., & Kastelein, J. J. P. (2022). Cholesteryl ester transfer protein inhibitors: from high-density lipoprotein cholesterol to low-density lipoprotein cholesterol lowering agents? *Cardiovascular Research*, *118*(14), 2919–2931. https://doi.org/10.1093/cvr/cvab350

O'Connell, E. M., & Lohoff, F. W. (2020). Proprotein convertase subtilisin/kexin type 9 (PCSK9) in the brain and relevance for neuropsychiatric disorders. *Frontiers in Neuroscience*, *14*, 609. doi.org/10.3389/fnins.2020.00609.

O'Donoghue, M. L., Fazio, S., Giugliano, R. P., Stroes, E. S. G., Kanevsky, E., Gouni-Berthold, I., Im, K., Lira Pineda, A., Wasserman, S. M., Češka, R., Ezhov, M. V., Jukema, J. W., Jensen, H. K., Tokgözoğlu, S. L., Mach, F., Huber, K., Sever, P. S., Keech, A. C., Pedersen, T. R., & Sabatine, M. S. (2019). Lipoprotein(a), PCSK9 inhibition, and cardiovascular risk. *Circulation*, *139*(12), 1483–1492. https://doi.org/10.1161/CIRCULATIONAHA.118.037184

O'Donoghue, M. L., Giugliano, R. P., Wiviott, S. D., Atar, D., Keech, A., Kuder, J. F., Im, K., Murphy, S. A., Flores-Arredondo, J. H., López, J. A. G., Elliott-Davey, M., Wang, B., Monsalvo, M. L., Abbasi, S., & Sabatine, M. S. (2022). Long-term evolocumab in patients with established atherosclerotic cardiovascular disease. *Circulation*, *146*(15), 1109–1119. doi.org/10.1161/CIRCULA TIONAHA.122.061620.

Ossoli, A., Neufeld, E. B., Thacker, S. G., Vaisman, B., Pryor, M., Freeman, L. A., Brantner, C. A., Baranova, I., Francone, N. O., Demosky, S. J., Jr, Vitali, C., Locatelli, M., Abbate, M., Zoja, C., Franceschini, G., Calabresi, L., & Remaley, A. T. (2016). Lipoprotein X causes renal disease in LCAT deficiency. *PloS one*, *11*(2), e0150083. https://doi.org/10.1371/journal.pone.0150083

Packard, C. J., Boren, J., & Taskinen, M. R. (2020). Causes and consequences of hypertriglyceridemia. *Frontiers in Endocrinology*, *11*, 252. doi.org/10.3389/fendo.2020.00252.

Pahlavani H. A. (2023). Exercise therapy to prevent and treat Alzheimer's disease. *Frontiers in Aging Neuroscience*, *15*, 1243869. https://doi.org/10.3389/fnagi.2023.1243869

Papotti, B., Adorni, M. P., Marchi, C., Zimetti, F., Ronda, N., Panighel, G., Lupo, M. G., Vilella, A., Giuliani, D., Ferri, N., & Bernini, F. (2022). PCSK9 affects astrocyte cholesterol metabolism and reduces neuron cholesterol supplying in vitro: Potential implications in Alzheimer's disease. *International Journal of Molecular Sciences, 23*(20), 12192. doi.org/10.3390/ijms232012192.

Pati, S., Irfan, W., Jameel, A., Ahmed, S., & Shahid, R. K. (2023). Obesity and cancer: A current overview of epidemiology, pathogenesis, outcomes, and management. *Cancers, 15*(2), 485. https://doi.org/10.3390/cancers15020485

Pedersen T. R. (2016). The Success story of LDL cholesterol lowering. *Circulation Research, 118*(4), 721–731. doi.org/10.1161/CIRCRESAHA.115.306297.

Picard, C., Nilsson, N., Labonté, A., Auld, D., Rosa-Neto, P., , Ashton, N. J., Zetterberg, H., Blennow, K., Breitner, J. C. B., Villeneuve, S., Poirier, J., & PREVENT-AD research group (2022). Apolipoprotein B is a novel marker for early tau pathology in Alzheimer's disease. *Alzheimer's & Dementia. The Journal of the Alzheimer's Association, 18*(5), 875–887. doi.org/10.1002/alz.12442.

Post, A., Tsikas, D., & Bakker, S. J. L. (2019). Creatine is a conditionally essential nutrient in chronic kidney disease: A hypothesis and narrative literature review. *Nutrients, 11*(5), 1044. https://doi.org/10.3390/nu11051044

Räber, L., Ueki, Y., Otsuka, T., Losdat, S., Häner, J. D., Lonborg, J., Fahrni, G., Iglesias, J. F., van Geuns, R. J., Ondracek, A. S., Radu Juul Jensen, M. D., Zanchin, C., Stortecky, S., Spirk, D., Siontis, G. C. M., Saleh, L., Matter, C. M., Daemen, J., Mach, F., Heg, D., ... PACMAN-AMI collaborators (2022). Effect of alirocumab added to high-intensity statin therapy on coronary atherosclerosis in patients with acute myocardial infarction: The PACMAN-AMI Randomized Clinical Trial. *JAMA, 327*(18), 1771–1781. https://doi.org/10.1001/jama.2022.5218

Raitakari, O., Kartiosuo, N., Pahkala, K., Hutri-Kähönen, N., Bazzano, L. A., Chen, W., Urbina, E. M., Jacobs, D. R., Jr, Sinaiko, A., Steinberger, J., Burns, T., Daniels, S. R., Venn, A., Woo, J. G., Dwyer, T., Juonala, M., & Viikari, J. (2023). Lipoprotein(a) in youth and prediction of major cardiovascular outcomes in adulthood. *Circulation, 147*(1), 23–31. doi.org/10.1161/CIRCULATIONAHA.122.060667

Raji, C., Dolatshahi, M., Rahmani, F., Commean, P., Nguyen, C., Ippolito, J., & Benzinger, T. (2023). Body Mass Index, but not visceral abdominal bbesity and insulin resistance, negatively impacts white matter microstructure in midlife. *Alzheimer's & Dementia.* 19. 10.1002/alz.075829.

Raufman J. P. (1996). Bioactive peptides from lizard venoms. *Regulatory Peptides, 61*(1), 1–18. https://doi.org/10.1016/0167-0115(96)00135-8

Raut, S., Bhalerao, A., Powers, M., Gonzalez, M., Mancuso, S., & Cucullo, L. (2023). Hypometabolism, Alzheimer's disease, and possible therapeutic targets: An overview. *Cells, 12*(16), 2019. doi.org/10.3390/cells12162019.

Ray, K. K., Troquay, R. P. T., Visseren, F. L. J., Leiter, L. A., Scott Wright, R., Vikarunnessa, S., Talloczy, Z., Zang, X., Maheux, P., Lesogor, A., & Landmesser, U. (2023). Long-term efficacy and safety of inclisiran in patients with high cardiovascular risk and elevated LDL cholesterol (ORION-3): results from the 4-year open-label extension of the ORION-1 trial. *The Lancet. Diabetes & Endocrinology, 11*(2), 109–119. https://doi.org/10.1016/S2213-

8587(22)00353-9

Richards, C. E., & Obaid, D. R. (2019). Low-dose radiation advances in coronary computed tomography angiography in the diagnosis of coronary artery disease. *Current Cardiology Reviews*, *15*(4), 304–315. https://doi.org/10.2174/1573403X15666190222163737

Rosoff, D. B., Bell, A. S., Jung, J., Wagner, J., Mavromatis, L. A., & Lohoff, F. W. (2022). Mendelian randomization study of PCSK9 and HMG-CoA reductase inhibition and cognitive function. *Journal of the American College of Cardiology*, *80*(7), 653–662. doi.org/10.1016/j.jacc.2022.05.041.

Ruder, S., Mansfield, B., Immelman, A. R., Varki, N., Miu, P., Raal, F., & Tsimikas, S. (2022). Lp(a), oxidized phospholipids and oxidation-specific epitopes are increased in subjects with keloid formation. *Lipids in Health and Disease*, *21*(1), 113. doi.org/10.1186/s12944-022-01720-z

Ruder, S., Mansfield, B., Immelman, A. R., Varki, N., Miu, P., Raal, F., & Tsimikas, S. (2022). Lp(a), oxidized phospholipids and oxidation-specific epitopes are increased in subjects with keloid formation. *Lipids in Health and Disease*, *21*(1), 113. https://doi.org/10.1186/s12944-022-01720-z

Ryan, T. E., Torres, M. J., Lin, C. T., Clark, A. H., Brophy, P. M., Smith, C. A., Smith, C. D., Morris, E. M., Thyfault, J. P., & Neufer, P. D. (2024). High-dose atorvastatin therapy progressively decreases skeletal muscle mitochondrial respiratory capacity in humans. *JCI Insight*, *9*(4), e174125. doi.org/10.1172/jci.insight.174125

Sakamoto, A., Cornelissen, A., Sato, Y., Mori, M., Kawakami, R., Kawai, K., Ghosh, S. K. B., Xu, W., Abebe, B. G., Dikongue, A., Kolodgie, F. D., Virmani, R., & Finn, A. V. (2022). Vulnerable plaque in patients with acute coronary syndrome: Identification, importance, and management. *US Cardiology Review*, *16*, e01. doi.org/10.15420/usc.2021.22

Sato, N., & Morishita, R. (2015). The roles of lipid and glucose metabolism in modulation of β-amyloid, tau, and neurodegeneration in the pathogenesis of Alzheimer disease. *Frontiers in Aging Neuroscience*, *7*, 199. doi.org/10.3389/fnagi.2015.00199.

Sato, Y., Suzuki, I., Nakamura, T., Bernier, F., Aoshima, K., & Oda, Y. (2012). Identification of a new plasma biomarker of Alzheimer's disease using metabolomics technology. *Journal of Lipid Research*, *53*(3), 567–576. doi.org/10.1194/jlr.M022376.

Schultz, B. G., Patten, D. K., & Berlau, D. J. (2018). The role of statins in both cognitive impairment and protection against dementia: a tale of two mechanisms. *Translational Neurodegeneration*, *7*, 5. doi.org/10.1186/s40035-018-0110-3.

Schwartz, G. G., Szarek, M., Bittner, V. A., Diaz, R., Goodman, S. G., Jukema, J. W., Landmesser, U., López-Jaramillo, P., Manvelian, G., Pordy, R., Scemama, M., Sinnaeve, P. R., White, H. D., Gabriel Steg, P., & ODYSSEY Outcomes Committees and Investigators (2021). Lipoprotein(a) and benefit of PCSK9 inhibition in patients with nominally controlled LDL cholesterol. *Journal of the American College of Cardiology*, *78*(5), 421–433. https://doi.org/10.1016/j.jacc.2021.04.102

Scott Kiss, R., & Sniderman, A. (2017). Shunts, channels and lipoprotein endosomal traffic: A new model of cholesterol homeostasis in the hepatocyte. Journal of Biomedical Research, 31(2), 95–107. https://doi.org/10.7555/JBR.31.20160139

Seidah, N., & Prat, A. (2022). The Multifaceted biology of PCSK9. *Endocrine Reviews*, *12*(43), 558–582. doi: 10.1210/endrev/bnab035.

Sharma, N., Ooi, J. L., Ong, J., & Newman, D. (2015). The use of fenofibrate in the management of patients with diabetic retinopathy: An evidence-based review. *Australian Family physician*, *44*(6), 367–370.

She, J., Tuerhongjiang, G., Guo, M., Liu, J., Hao, X., Guo, L., Liu, N., Xi, W., Zheng, T., Du, B., Lou, B., Gao, X., Yuan, X., Yu, Y., Zhang, Y., Gao, F., Zhuo, X., Xiong, Y., Zhang, X., Yu, J., ... Wu, Y. (2024). Statins aggravate insulin resistance through reduced blood glucagon-like peptide-1 levels in a microbiota-dependent manner. *Cell Metabolism*, *36*(2), 408–421.e5. doi.org/10.1016/j.cmet.2023.12.027

Sherratt, S. C. R., Juliano, R. A., & Mason, R. P. (2020). Eicosapentaenoic acid (EPA) has optimal chain length and degree of unsaturation to inhibit oxidation of small dense LDL and membrane cholesterol domains as compared to related fatty acids in vitro. *Biomembranes*, *1862*(7), 183254. doi.org/10.1016/j.bbamem.2020.183254

Shiyovich, A., Berman, A. N., Besser, S. A., Biery, D. W., Kaur, G., Divakaran, S., Singh, A., Huck, D. M., Weber, B., Plutzky, J., Di Carli, M. F., Nasir, K., Cannon, C., Januzzi, J. L., Bhatt, D. L., & Blankstein, R. (2024). Association of lipoprotein (a) and standard modifiable cardiovascular risk factors with incident myocardial infarction: The mass general Brigham lp(a) registry. *Journal of the American Heart Association*, *13*(10), e034493. doi.org/10.1161/JAHA.123.034493

Shu, X., Wu, J., Zhang, T., Ma, X., Du, Z., Xu, J., You, J., Wang, L., Chen, N., Luo, M., & Wu, J. (2022). Statin-induced geranylgeranyl pyrophosphate depletion promotes PCSK9-dependent adipose insulin resistance. *Nutrients*, *14*(24), 5314. doi.org/10.3390/nu14245314.

Simeone, P. G., Vadini, F., Tripaldi, R., Liani, R., Ciotti, S., Di Castelnuovo, A., Cipollone, F., & Santilli, F. (2021). Sex-specific association of endogenous PCSK9 with memory function in elderly subjects at high cardiovascular risk. *Frontiers in Aging Neuroscience*, *13*, 632-655. doi.org/10.3389/fnagi.2021.632655.

Singh, M., Kapoor, A., & Bhatnagar, A. (2021). Physiological and pathological roles of aldose reductase. *Metabolites*, *11*(10), 655. https://doi.org/10.3390/metabo11100655

Sinzinger, H., & O'Grady, J. (2004). Professional athletes suffering from familial hypercholesterolemia rarely tolerate statin treatment because of muscular problems. *British Journal of Clinical Pharmacology*, *57*(4), 525–528. doi.org/10.1111/j.1365-2125.2003.02044.x

Sinzinger, H., & O'Grady, J. (2004). Professional athletes suffering from familial hypercholesterolaemia rarely tolerate statin treatment because of muscular problems. *British Journal of Clinical Pharmacology*, *57*(4), 525–528. doi.org/10.1111/j.1365-2125.2003.02044.x.

Sittiwet, C., Simonen, P., Nissinen, M. J., Gylling, H., & Strandberg, T. E. (2018). Serum noncholesterol sterols in Alzheimer's disease: The Helsinki businessmen study. *Translational Research: The Journal of Laboratory and Clinical Medicine*, *202*, 120–128. doi.org/10.1016/j.trsl.2018.07.002.

Skogsberg, J., Dicker, A., Rydén, M., Åström, G., Nilsson, R., Bhuiyan, H., Vitols, S., Mairal, A., Langin, D., Alberts, P., Walum, E., Tegnér, J., Hamsten, A., Arner, P., & Björkegren, J. (2008). ApoB100-LDL acts as a metabolic signal from liver to peripheral fat causing inhibition of lipolysis in adipocytes. *PLoS ONE*, *3*(11), e3771. doi.org/10.1371/journal.pone.0003771

Song, J. D., Alves, T. C., Befroy, D. E., Perry, R. J., Mason, G. F., Zhang, X. M., Munk, A., Zhang, Y., Zhang, D., Cline, G. W., Rothman, D. L., Petersen, K. F., & Shulman, G. I. (2020). Dissociation of muscle insulin resistance from alterations in mitochondrial substrate preference. *Cell Metabolism*, *32*(5), 726–735.e5. https://doi.org/10.1016/j.cmet.2020.09.008

SPRINT Research Group, Lewis, C. E., Fine, L. J., Beddhu, S., Cheung, A. K., Cushman, W. C., Cutler, J. A., Evans, G. W., Johnson, K. C., Kitzman, D. W., Oparil, S., Rahman, M., Reboussin, D. M., Rocco, M. V., Sink, K. M., Snyder, J. K., Whelton, P. K., Williamson, J. D., Wright, J. T., Jr, & Ambrosius, W. T. (2021). Final report of a trial of intensive versus standard blood-pressure control. *The New England Journal of Medicine*, *384*(20), 1921–1930. https://doi.org/10.1056/NEJMoa1901281

Stegman, B., Shao, M., Nicholls, S. J., Elshazly, M., Cho, L., King, P., Kapadia, S., Tuzcu, M., Nissen, S. E., & Puri, R. (2016). Coronary atheroma progression rates in men and women following high-intensity statin therapy: A pooled analysis of REVERSAL, ASTEROID and SATURN. *Atherosclerosis*, *254*, 78–84. https://doi.org/10.1016/j.atherosclerosis.2016.09.059

Sumner, A. E., Finley, K. B., Genovese, D. J., Criqui, M. H., & Boston, R. C. (2005). Fasting triglyceride and the triglyceride-HDL cholesterol ratio are not markers of insulin resistance in African Americans. *Archives of Internal Medicine*, *165*(12), 1395–1400. https://doi.org/10.1001/archinte.165.12.1395

Svilaas, T., Klemsdal, T. O., Bogsrud, M. P., Græsdal, A., Vesterbekkmo, E. K., Asprusten, E. A., Langslet, G., & Retterstøl, K. (2022). High levels of lipoprotein(a): Assessment and treatment. *Tidsskrift for den Norske laegeforening: Tidsskrift for praktisk medicin, ny raekke*, *142*(1), 10.4045/tidsskr.21.0800. https://doi.org/10.4045/tidsskr.21.0800

Taageby Nielsen, S., Mohr Lytsen, R., Strandkjær, N., Juul Rasmussen, I., Sillesen, A. S., Vøgg, R. O. B., Axelsson Raja, A., Nordestgaard, B. G., Kamstrup, P. R., Iversen, K., Bundgaard, H., Tybjærg-Hansen, A., & Frikke-Schmidt, R.

(2023). Significance of lipids, lipoproteins, and apolipoproteins during the first 14-16 months of life. *European Heart Journal*, *44*(42), 4408–4418. https://doi.org/10.1093/eurheartj/ehad547

Trinder, M., Zekavat, S. M., Uddin, M. M., Pampana, A., & Natarajan, P. (2021). Apolipoprotein B is an insufficient explanation for the risk of coronary disease associated with lipoprotein(a). *Cardiovascular Research*, *117*(5), 1245–1247. doi.org/10.1093/cvr/cvab060

Valenti, V., Ó Hartaigh, B., Heo, R., Cho, I., Schulman-Marcus, J., Gransar, H., Truong, Q. A., Shaw, L. J., Knapper, J., Kelkar, A. A., Sandesara, P., Lin, F. Y., Sciarretta, S., Chang, H. J., Callister, T. Q., & Min, J. K. (2015). A 15-year warranty period for asymptomatic individuals without coronary artery calcium: A prospective follow-up of 9,715 individuals. *JACC Cardiovascular Imaging*, *8*(8), 900–909. doi.org/10.1016/j.jcmg.2015.01.025

Varghese, J., & Dakhode, S. (2022). Effects of alcohol consumption on various systems of the human body: A systematic review. *Cureus*, *14*(10), e30057. https://doi.org/10.7759/cureus.30057

Varma, V. R., Büşra Lüleci, H., Oommen, A. M., Varma, S., Blackshear, C. T., Griswold, M. E., An, Y., Roberts, J. A., O'Brien, R., Pletnikova, O., Troncoso, J. C., Bennett, D. A., Çakır, T., Legido-Quigley, C., & Thambisetty, M. (2021). Abnormal brain cholesterol homeostasis in Alzheimer's disease-a targeted metabolomic and transcriptomic study. *NPJ Aging and Mechanisms of Disease*, *7*(1), 11. doi.org/10.1038/s41514-021-00064-9.

Vasunilashorn, S., Crimmins, E. M., Kim, J. K., Winking, J., Gurven, M., Kaplan, H., & Finch, C. E. (2010). Blood lipids, infection, and inflammatory markers in the Tsimane of Bolivia. *American Journal of Human Biology: The Official Journal of the Human Biology Council*, *22*(6), 731–740. doi.org/10.1002/ajhb.21074

Vesterbekkmo, E. K., Aksetøy, I. A., Follestad, T., Nilsen, H. O., Hegbom, K., Wisløff, U., Wiseth, R., & Madssen, E. (2023). High-intensity interval training induces beneficial effects on coronary atheromatous plaques: a randomized trial. *European Journal of Preventive Cardiology*, *30*(5), 384–392. doi.org/10.1093/eurjpc/zwac309

Vilella, A., Bodria, M., Papotti, B., Zanotti, I., Zimetti, F., Remaggi, G., Elviri, L., Potì, F., Ferri, N., Lupo, M. G., Panighel, G., Daini, E., Vandini, E., Zoli, M., Giuliani, D., & Bernini, F. (2024). PCSK9 ablation attenuates Aβ pathology, neuroinflammation and cognitive dysfunctions in 5XFAD mice. *Brain, Behavior, and Immunity*, *115*, 517–534. https://doi.org/10.1161/JAHA.118.010838

Virani, S. S., Newby, L. K., Arnold, S. V., Bittner, V., Brewer, L. C., Demeter, S. H., Dixon, D. L., Fearon, W. F., Hess, B., Johnson, H. M., Kazi, D. S., Kolte, D., Kumbhani, D. J., LoFaso, J., Mahtta, D., Mark, D. B., Minissian, M., Navar, A. M., Patel, A. R., Piano, M. R., ... Williams, M. S. (2023). 2023 AHA/ACC/ACCP/ASPC/NLA/PCNA Guideline for the management of patients with chronic coronary disease: A report of the American Heart Association/American College of Cardiology Joint Committee on clinical practice guidelines. *Circulation*, *148*(9), e9–e119. doi.org/10.1161/CIR.0000000000001168.

Wang, H., He, S., Wang, J., An, Y., Wang, X., Li, G., & Gong, Q. (2023). Hyperinsulinemia and plasma glucose level independently associated with all-cause and cardiovascular mortality in Chinese people without diabetes-A post-hoc analysis of the 30-year follow-up of Da Qing diabetes and IGT study. *Diabetes Res Clinical Practice*. 1(195). doi: 10.1016/j.diabres.2022.110199

Wang, L., Zheng, Z., Zhu, L., Meng, L., Liu, H., Wang, K., Chen, J., Li, P., & Yang, H. (2022). Geranylgeranyl pyrophosphate depletion by statins compromises skeletal muscle insulin sensitivity. *Journal of Cachexia, Sarcopenia and Muscle*, *13*(6), 2697–2711. doi.org/10.1002/jcsm.13061

Wang, Y., Spolitu, S., Zadroga, J. A., Sarecha, A. K., & Ozcan, L. (2022). Hepatocyte Rap1a contributes to obesity- and statin-associated hyperglycemia. *Cell Reports*, *40*(8), 111259. doi.org/10.1016/j.celrep.2022.111259.

Wheeler, S., & Sillence, D. (2020) Niemann-Pick type C disease: Cellular pathology and pharmacotherapy. *Journal of Neurochemistry, 153,* 674-692. doi: 10.1111/jnc.14895.

Wilkins, J. T., Li, R. C., Sniderman, A., Chan, C., & Lloyd-Jones, D. M. (2016). Discordance between Apolipoprotein B and LDL-cholesterol in young adults predicts coronary artery calcification: The CARDIA Study. *Journal of the American College of Cardiology*, *67*(2), 193–201. doi.org/10.1016/j.jacc.2015.10.055

Willeit, P., Ridker, P. M., Nestel, P. J., Simes, J., Tonkin, A. M., Pedersen, T. R., Schwartz, G. G., Olsson, A. G., Colhoun, H. M., Kronenberg, F., Drechsler, C., Wanner, C., Mora, S., Lesogor, A., & Tsimikas, S. (2018). Baseline and on-statin treatment lipoprotein(a) levels for prediction of cardiovascular events: Individual patient-data meta-analysis of statin outcome trials. *Lancet (London, England)*, *392*(10155), 1311–1320. doi.org/10.1016/S0140-6736(18)31652-0

Williams, L., Rhodes, K. S., Karmally, W., Welstead, L. A., Alexander, L., Sutton, L., & patients and families living with FCS (2018). Familial chylomicronemia syndrome: Bringing to life dietary recommendations throughout the life span. *Journal of Clinical Lipidology*, *12*(4), 908–919. https://doi.org/10.1016/j.jacl.2018.04.010

Woudberg, N. J., Pedretti, S., Lecour, S., Schulz, R., Vuilleumier, N., James, R. W., & Frias, M. A. (2018). Pharmacological intervention to modulate HDL: What do we target? *Frontiers in Pharmacology*, *8*, 989. https://doi.org/10.3389/fphar.2017.00989

Xie, B., Shi, X., Xing, Y., & Tang, Y. (2020). Association between atherosclerosis and Alzheimer's disease: A systematic review and meta-analysis. *Brain and Behavior*, *10*(4), e01601. doi.org/10.1002/brb3.1601.

Yanai, H., Adachi, H., Hakoshima, M., & Katsuyama, H. (2023). Postprandial hyperlipidemia: Its pathophysiology, diagnosis, atherogenesis, and treatments. *International Journal of Molecular Sciences*, *24*(18), 13942. doi.org/10.3390/ijms241813942.

Yao, H., Pang, Y., Chen, Y., Si, N., Wu, C., Wang, Z., & Ren, Y. (2023). Association between interleukin-6 gene polymorphism and severity of coronary artery disease in patients with diabetes. *Diabetes, Metabolic Syndrome and Obesity: Targets and Therapy*, *16*, 3599–3608. https://doi.org/10.2147/DMSO.S427873

Yassine, H. N., Braskie, M. N., Mack, W. J., Castor, K. J., Fonteh, A. N., Schneider, L. S., Harrington, M. G., & Chui, H. C. (2017). Association of docosahexaenoic acid supplementation with Alzheimer disease stage in apolipoprotein e ε4 carriers: A review. *JAMA Neurology*, *74*(3), 339–347. doi.org/10.1001/jamaneurol.2016.4899.

Youssef, A., Clark, J. R., Marcovina, S. M., Boffa, M. B., & Koschinsky, M. L. (2022). Apo(a) and ApoB interact noncovalently within hepatocytes: Implications for regulation of Lp(a) levels by modulation of ApoB secretion. *Arteriosclerosis, Thrombosis, and Vascular Biology*, *42*(3), 289–304. doi.org/10.1161/ATVBAHA.121.317335.

Yuyun, M. F., Khaw, K. T., Luben, R., Welch, A., Bingham, S., Day, N. E., Wareham, N. J., & European Prospective Investigation into Cancer in Norfolk (EPIC-Norfolk) population study (2004). Microalbuminuria independently predicts all-cause and cardiovascular mortality in a British population: The European Prospective Investigation into Cancer in Norfolk (EPIC-Norfolk) population study. *International Journal of Epidemiology*, *33*(1), 189–198. https://doi.org/10.1093/ije/dyh008

Zhang, J., & Liu, Q. (2015). Cholesterol metabolism and homeostasis in the brain. *Protein & Cell*, *6*(4), 254–264. doi.org/10.1007/s13238-014-0131-3.

Zheng, C., Andraski, A. B., Khoo, C., Furtado, J. D., & Sacks, F. M. (2024). Food intake suppresses apoB secretion and fractional catabolic rates in humans. *Arteriosclerosis, Thrombosis, and Vascular Biology*, *44*(2), 435–451. https://doi.org/10.1161/ATVBAHA.123.319769

Zhu, L., Fang, Y., Gao, B., Jin, X., Zheng, J., He, Y., & Huang, J. (2022). Effect of an increase in Lp(a) following statin therapy on cardiovascular prognosis in secondary prevention population of coronary artery disease. *BMC Cardiovascular Disorders*, *22*(1), 474. doi.org/10.1186/s12872-022-02932-y

Zhu, L., Fang, Y., Gao, B., Jin, X., Zheng, J., He, Y., & Huang, J. (2022). Effect of an increase in Lp(a) following statin therapy on cardiovascular prognosis in secondary prevention population of coronary artery disease. *BMC Cardiovascular Disorders*, *22*(1), 474. doi.org/10.1186/s12872-022-02932-y.

Zimerman, A., O'Donoghue, M., Ran, X., Im, K., Ott, B.F., Mach, F., Zavitz, K., Kurtz, C.E., Monsalvo, M.L., Wang, B., Atar, D., Keech, A., Sabatine, M.S., & Guigliano, R. (2023). Abstract 14714: Long-term neurocognitive safety of LCL-C lowering with evolocumab: Open-label extension data from FOURIER. *American Heart Association, 148*: A14714. https://doi.org/10.1161/circ.148.suppl_1.14714.

Made in the USA
Coppell, TX
31 January 2026